Tuberculosis: A Clinical Practice Guide

Authored by

Rafael Laniado-Laborín

Tuberculosis Clinic
Tijuana Mexico General Hospital
School of Medicine
Autonomous University of Baja California
Mexico

Tuberculosis: A Clinical Practice Guide

Author: Rafael Lani

ISBN (Online): 978-981-14-8851-1

ISBN (Print): 978-981-14-8849-8

ISBN (Paperback): 978-981-14-8850-4

need for a court order if at any point you breach any terms of this License Agreement. In no event will any delay or failure by Bentham Science Publishers in enforcing your compliance with this License Agreement constitute a waiver of any of its rights.

3. You acknowledge that you have read this License Agreement, and agree to be bound by its terms and conditions. To the extent that any other terms and conditions presented on any website of Bentham Science Publishers conflict with, or are inconsistent with, the terms and conditions set out in this License Agreement, you acknowledge that the terms and conditions set out in this License Agreement shall prevail.

Bentham Science Publishers Pte. Ltd.
80 Robinson Road #02-00
Singapore 068898
Singapore
Email: subscriptions@benthamscience.net

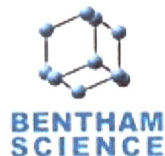

BENTHAM SCIENCE

CONTENTS

FOREWORD

Dr. Laniado Laborín has accumulated vast experience in various fields of Pulmonology and Public Health, specialties that he has practiced for 40 years, standing out, especially in tuberculosis and drug-resistant tuberculosis.

He has numerous publications on this topic, but, more than what is written, I would have to ponder his experience accumulated over the years treating patients with this ancient disease that science has not yet managed to control, much less eradicate. Many difficult patients have passed through the Tuberculosis Clinic of the General Hospital of Tijuana, especially those who suffer from drug-resistant forms of the disease, aggravated by the vulnerable conditions that are unfortunately so frequently associated, and to whom he has always devoted a full attention in terms of humanity and knowledge.

His teaching performance as a professor at the Autonomous University of Tijuana is nationally and internationally recognized for his knowledge and human qualities. Countless young doctors have rotated through his service, taking a clear perception of tuberculosis's reality, both from a scientific, social and human point of view.

He has published several books throughout his career, including Drug-resistant Tuberculosis, A Practical Guide, and La Tuberculosis en México.

The work to which we have been granted the honor of writing the prologue, Tuberculosis: A Clinical Practice Guide, displays throughout its 16 chapters a detailed and well-founded overview of the disease, from epidemiology, clinical aspects, diagnosis, and prevention, in addition to delving into particular aspects such as special situations and, of course, devotes several chapters to the medical treatment of sensitive and drug-resistant TB, surgical aspects and a difficult subject such as adverse reactions to anti-tuberculosis drugs. The 15 images of outstanding quality included in the chapter of radiologic diagnosis of tuberculosis are paradigmatic of various pulmonary, extrapulmonary, and disseminated TB situations. In the 24 tables of the work, various aspects are clearly and precisely summarized, such as first and second-line drugs, treatment, and retreatment schemes.

The author, showing off his proverbial modesty, directs his work to students and health personnel who are not experts in tuberculosis. After reading, which is enjoyable and shows the extensive experience of Dr. Laniado Laborín on the subject, I have concluded that the book goes beyond these objectives, as it provides throughout its 150 pages (expandable through of the excellent bibliography that proposes) a synthesis of the current state of the art on the disease, which will provide to those who assimilate them with the knowledge of an expert in tuberculosis.

So let us welcome this work for its quality and ease of reading, which will undoubtedly occupy a prominent place in the tuberculosis literature.

Domingo Palmero
Professor of Pneumology, University of Buenos Aires
Argentina

PREFACE

"Of all the forms of inequality, injustice in health care
is the most shocking and inhumane"
Martin Luther King Jr. (1929-1968)

Tuberculosis has accompanied human beings since time immemorial, and without a doubt, it is the disease of infectious origin that has caused the highest number of deaths in the history of humankind.

However, despite the extraordinary technological advances achieved in the last decade, tuberculosis continues to cause more than 10 million cases and 1.3 million deaths annually.

The reasons that explain this pandemic are multiple, mainly poverty and poor medical care (95% of cases and deaths occur in low-income countries); other contributing factors include infection by the human immunodeficiency virus, substance abuse and the emergence of drug-resistant tuberculosis.

An additional contributing factor is the little attention that has been paid to the disease in the training of health personnel, where maybe a couple of hours are dedicated to the subject in the curriculum of universities. This lack of attention results in insufficient knowledge of tuberculosis, with the consequent delay in diagnosis and the prescription of inadequate treatment.

This book aims to be a reference manual for the student and health personnel who are not an expert in tuberculosis, since it contains information on all topics related to the disease, including epidemiological, microbiological, clinical, diagnostic and treatment aspects, BCG vaccination and the control of tuberculosis infection in health facilities.

I hope this work is useful for my colleagues during their everyday practice and benefits our patients that suffer from tuberculosis.

CONSENT FOR PUBLICATION

Not applicable.

CONFLICT OF INTEREST

The author declares no conflict of interest, financial or otherwise.

ACKNOWLEDGEMENTS

Declared none.

Rafael Laniado-Laborín
Tuberculosis Clinic,
Tijuana General Hospital,
Mexico School of Medicine,
Autonomous University of Baja California,
Mexico
E-mail: rlaniado@uabc.edu.mx

DEDICATION

Dedicated to
My family for their patience and support, and our patients,
which through their suffering have taught us the best way to take care of them.

Tijuana, Mexico. August 2020.

CHAPTER 1

Tuberculosis Global Epidemiology

Abstract: Globally, tuberculosis is one of the top 10 overall causes of death, the leading cause of death from a single infectious agent, and the principal cause of death among subjects living with human immunodeficiency virus infection.

The United Nations and the World Health Organization (WHO) have set very ambitious goals for the period 2020-2035 that include a 95% reduction in the number of deaths and a 90% reduction in TB incidence by 2035 compared with 2015.

The WHO reported in 2018, an estimated 10 million incident cases of TB (global incidence rate: 133 cases per 10^5 population), and 1.2 million TB deaths, for a case fatality rate of 15.7%. Incidence rates vary widely among regions of the world; geographically, most TB cases in 2018 were in the WHO regions of South-East Asia (44%), Africa (24%) and the Western Pacific (18%).

Rifampin-resistant (RR-TB) or multidrug-resistant TB (MDR-TB) in 2018 occurred in an estimated half a million cases, and accounted for 3.4% of all new cases and 18% of previously treated cases; an estimated 230,000 persons died of either RR or MDR-TB (case fatality rate: 41%).

Almost a quarter of the world population (1.7 billion people or 23%) are estimated to have latent TB infection and therefore are at risk of developing active TB during their lifetime.

Progress toward global TB elimination during 2018 was very modest, as it has occurred in recent years, and if kept at this current pace, the global targets for the period 2020-2035 will not be accomplished.

Keywords: Epidemiology, Incidence, MDR-TB, Mortality, Tuberculosis, XDR-TB.

INTRODUCTION

Tuberculosis (TB) has affected humans for most of its history and continues to do so even though we have had an effective pharmacological treatment for more than 70 years [1]. TB is a leading cause of death among adults in the most productive age groups, and even those that have been cured can be left with significant irreversible sequelae that will substantially affect their quality of life [2].

Globally, tuberculosis is one of the top 10 overall causes of death, the leading cause of death from a single infectious agent, and the principal cause of death among subjects living with human immunodeficiency virus infection, causing approximately 40% of deaths in this population group [3].

The United Nations (UN) and the World Health Organization (WHO) have set very ambitious goals for the period 2020-2035 (Table **1**) that include a 95% reduction in the number of deaths and a 90% reduction in TB incidence by 2035 compared with 2015 [4, 5].

Table 1. The End TB Strategy. A world free of TB: zero deaths, disease and suffering due to tuberculosis*.

Indicators	2020	2025	2030	2035
Percentage reduction in the absolute number of TB deaths (compared with 2015 baseline)	35%	75%	90%	95%
Percentage reduction in the TB incidence rate (compared with 2015 baseline)	20%	50%	80%	90%
Percentage of TB-affected households experiencing catastrophic costs due to TB	0%	0%	0%	0%

*modified from WHO Global Tuberculosis Report 2018 [9].

A Stop TB Partnership target is that by the year 2050, the global incidence of active TB will be less than one case per million population per year. The components of the Stop TB Strategy are:

1. Pursue high-quality DOTS expansion and enhancement.
2. Address TB-HIV, MDR-TB, and the needs of poor and vulnerable populations.
3. Contribute to health system strengthening based on primary health care.
4. Engage all care providers.
5. Empower people with TB, and communities through partnership.
6. Enable and promote research.

TUBERCULOSIS STATISTICS

TB incidence has never been measured at a country level, since this would require long term prospective studies, including large population cohorts (hundreds of thousands) with very high costs and challenging logistics. As a proxy of real incidence, TB incidence is estimated from case reports included in routine surveillance systems. Unfortunately, in many countries, surveillance systems cannot provide an adequate measure of TB incidence because of underreporting or underdiagnosis of cases [6].

Incidence rates vary widely among regions of the world (Table **2**). The lowest rates (<10 per 10^5) are reported from high-income countries including most countries from Western Europe, Canada, the United States, Australia, and New Zealand; most countries in the Americas (the WHO region with the lowest TB burden) have rates <50 per 10^5, although some countries like Haiti (181 per 10^5), Bolivia (111 per 10^5), and Peru (116 per 10^5) still have very high rates [7]. The countries with the highest rates are mostly located in Africa.

Table 2. Estimated number of incident tuberculosis (TB) cases, incidence, and percentage of deaths among all TB cases*.

WHO Region	No. Cases (×1000)	Incidence (Per 10^5)	Fatality Rate (%)
Global (all regions)	10,000	133	15.7
African	2,480	237	26.8
Americas	282	28	8.5
Eastern Mediterranean	771	113	11.9
European	273	30	10.6
South-East Asia	4,440	226	15.0
Western Pacific	1,800	94	5.4

*modified from WHO Global Tuberculosis Report, 2018 [9].

Geographically, most TB cases in 2018 were in the WHO regions of South-East Asia (44%), Africa (24%), and the Western Pacific (18%) [8]. Eight countries account for two-thirds of the world cases: India (27%), China (9%), Indonesia (8%), the Philippines (6%), Pakistan (5%), Nigeria (4%), Bangladesh (4%) and South Africa (3%). On the other hand, only 3% of the global cases are reported by the WHO European Region and 3% by the WHO Americas region [7, 9].

The WHO reported for the year 2018, an estimated 10 million (range 9.0-11.1 million) incident cases of TB (global rate: 133 cases per 10^5population), and 1.2 million TB deaths (range 1.1 to 1.3 million [8]. This represents a reduction of 1.8% and 3.9% in incident TB cases and TB deaths, respectively, in comparison with the year 2016; 920,000 (9%) of the incident cases and an estimated 300,000 deaths (case fatality rate 32.6%) occurred among persons living with HIV. Of the estimated 10 million cases, there were 5.8 million men, 3.2 million women, and 1 million children. Ninety percent of the cases are reported in adults (≥15 years), and, as mentioned, 9% occurred in people living with HIV, 72% of those living in Africa [9].

Rifampin-resistant (RR-TB) or multidrug-resistant TB (MDR-TB) occurred in an estimated half a million cases (range 417,000-556,000) in 2018, which constitutes

5.6% of all cases. RR/MDR-TB accounted for 3.4% and 18% of new and previously treated cases, respectively, in 2018; an estimated 230,000 persons died of either RR or MDR-TB (case fatality rate: 41%) [9]. Among the RR-TB cases, 78% were MDR [8]; of the MDR-TB cases, 8.5% ($CI_{95\%}$ 6.2-11%) were estimated to have extensively drug-resistant TB, also known as XDR-TB. Three countries accounted for almost half of the world cases of RR/MDR-TB: India (24%), China (13%), and the Russian Federation (10%). Although the overall incidence of TB in the WHO European region was only 30 per 10^5, the proportion of TB cases with RR or MDR-TB in this region (40%) was much higher than that in all the other five regions (range: 3.6%–6.3%) [9].

Almost a quarter of the world population (1.7 billion people or 23%) are estimated to have latent TB infection (LTBI) and therefore are at risk of developing active TB during their lifetime, become infectious, and transmit the disease [10].

Achieving the targets of the End TB strategy (Table **1**) for a reduction in TB cases and deaths set for 2020 and 2025 will require to accelerate the current annual decline from 1.5% per year in 2015 to 4-5% per year by 2020, and by 10% per year by 2025. The global proportion of people who die from TB (case fatality ratio) needs to be reduced from 15.7% in 2017 to 10% by 2020 and 6.5% by 2025. This reduction in rates will only be possible if all those with TB can access high-quality health services for early diagnosis and effective treatment.

Reaching the 2030 and 2035 targets will require an average acceleration of the decline rate of 17% per year. Such acceleration will depend on technological developments that could substantially reduce the risk of progression to an active disease of 1.7 billion people with LTBI through an effective post-exposure vaccine [11] or a concise, effective, and safe treatment for LTBI [1, 6].

Despite advances in treatment and prevention, tuberculosis is one of the leading causes of morbidity and mortality and the leading cause of death from an infectious disease globally.

Tuberculosis ceased to be an essential public health issue in economically developed countries as the main determinants of disease -extreme poverty, severe malnutrition, and overcrowding- gradually disappeared. Some public health experts declared that "virtual elimination of tuberculosis was in sight" [12].

Although the development of antibiotic resistance due to *M. tuberculosis* was reported almost immediately after the introduction of the first effective regimen in the treatment of tuberculosis in 1944 with streptomycin, the effectiveness of regimens consisting of a combination of several antimicrobials in the treatment of tuberculosis during the decades of the 50's and 60's, brought as a consequence, the lack of interest in the development of new anti-tuberculosis drugs; 40 years had to pass between the introduction of rifampicin in the 1960s and the development of two new drugs, bedaquiline and delamanid in the 2010s [13].

However, drug resistance is only one of the factors that favor the persistence of tuberculosis as a serious public health problem. Extreme poverty and co-infection with HIV in economically underdeveloped regions are a very significant contributing factor. Globalization has improved the mobility of the population but also the transmission of tuberculosis.

The control of tuberculosis will require a comprehensive approach to tackle the disease's socio-cultural determinants in combination with scientific advances in diagnosis [14] and treatment [15] if the disease is to be eradicated one day.

REFERENCES

[1]   MacNeil A, Glaziou P, Sismanidis C, Maloney S, Floyd K. Global epidemiology of tuberculosis and progress toward achieving global targets - 2017. MMWR Morb Mortal Wkly Rep 2019; 68(11): 263-6.
[http://dx.doi.org/10.15585/mmwr.mm6811a3] [PMID: 30897077]

[2]   Miller TL, McNabb SJ, Hilsenrath P, Pasipanodya J, Weis SE. Personal and societal health quality lost to tuberculosis. PLoS One 2009; 4(4): e5080.
[http://dx.doi.org/10.1371/journal.pone.0005080] [PMID: 19352424]

[3]   Gupta RK, Lucas SB, Fielding KL, Lawn SD. Prevalence of tuberculosis in post-mortem studies of HIV-infected adults and children in resource-limited settings: a systematic review and meta-analysis. AIDS 2015; 29(15): 1987-2002.
[http://dx.doi.org/10.1097/QAD.0000000000000802] [PMID: 26266773]

[4]   UN United Nations. Sustainable development goals New York, NY: United Nations 2016.
https://sustainabledevelopment.un.org

[5]   WHO World Health Organization. The end TB strategy Geneva, Switzerland: World Health Organization 2015. https://www.who.int/tb/strategy/ end-tb/en/

[6]   Glaziou P, Sismanidis C, Floyd K, Raviglione M, Raviglione M. Global epidemiology of tuberculosis. Cold Spring Harb Perspect Med 2014; 5(2): a017798.
[http://dx.doi.org/10.1101/cshperspect.a017798] [PMID: 25359550]

[7]   OPS. Organización Panamericana de la Salud 2018. Tuberculosis en las Américas 2018. Washington, DC: OPS, 2018. Número de documento: OPS/CDE/18-036

[8]   WHO. Global tuberculosis report 2019. Geneva: World Health Organization; 2019. Licence: CC BY-NC-SA 3.0 IGO.

[9]   WHO. World Health Organization Global tuberculosis report 2018. Geneva, Switzerland: World Health Organization 2018.

[10] Houben RM, Dodd PJ. The global burden of latent tuberculosis infection: a re-estimation using mathematical modelling. PLoS Med 2016; 13(10): e1002152.
[http://dx.doi.org/10.1371/journal] [PMID: 1002152]

[11] Tait DR, Hatherill M, Van Der Meeren O, *et al.* Final Analysis of a Trial of M72/AS01$_E$ Vaccine to Prevent Tuberculosis. N Engl J Med 2019; 381(25): 2429-39.
[http://dx.doi.org/10.1056/NEJMoa1909953] [PMID: 31661198]

[12]   Castro KG, LoBue P. Bridging implementation, knowledge, and ambition gaps to eliminate tuberculosis in the United States and globally. Emerg Infect Dis 2011; 17(3): 337-42.
[http://dx.doi.org/10.3201/eid1703.110031] [PMID: 21392421]

[13]   Armocida E, Martini .*M Tuberculosis*: a timeless challenge for medicine. J Prev Med Hyg 2020; 61(2): E143-7.
[http://dx.doi.org/10.15167/2421-4248/jpmh2020.61.2.1402] [PMID: 32802997]

[14]   WHO consolidated guidelines on tuberculosis. Module 3: diagnosis – rapid diagnostics for tuberculosis detection. Geneva: World Health Organization; 2020. Licence: CC BY-NC-SA 3.0 IGO.

[15]   WHO consolidated guidelines on tuberculosis. Module 4: treatment - drug-resistant tuberculosis treatment. Geneva: World Health Organization; 2020. Licence: CC BY-NC-SA 3.0 IGO.

CHAPTER 2

Microbiology of Tuberculosis

Abstract: *Mycobacterium tuberculosis* (MTB) is the primary etiological agent of tuberculosis in humans (since the disease may be due to other mycobacteria of the MTB complex such as *M. bovis*). It belongs to the order of the *Actinomycetales* and the *Mycobacteriaceae* family. It is a bacillus that lacks capsule or flagella and does not produce spores or toxins; it measures 0.5 by four microns. Its generation time is prolonged (up to 24 hours). It is an aerobic bacillus that, if necessary, can persist under anaerobic conditions.

It has a cell wall of extremely complex composition, with great strength and thickness, constituted up to 60% by lipids, generally known as mycolic acids that form complexes with polysaccharides such as arabinogalactan and peptidoglycan; these lipids determine their resistance to discoloration by alcohol-acid after they have been stained with carbol fuchsin (hence the term acid-fast bacilli acid or AFB). A distinctive feature of the MTB cell wall is its content of N-glycolimuranic acid instead of N-acetylmuramic acid found in most bacteria.

The unusual cell wall of MTB also allows it to survive initially in the macrophage. The cell wall also constitutes a robust and highly impermeable barrier to harmful compounds and drugs. MTB can sense when the local tissue conditions are inadequate for survival (low oxygen tension and nutrient depletion), as in the macrophages and granulomas, responding by the activation of a dormant state, in which the bacilli stop multiplying, down-regulates its metabolism and activates anaerobic metabolism.

Keywords: Acid-fast bacilli, Granulomas, *Mycobacterium tuberculosis*, Mycolic acids.

INTRODUCTION

The *Mycobacterium Tuberculosis* Complex (MTC)

Members of the MTC are bacteria that share a genetically identical 16SrRNA sequence and a greater 99.9% nucleotide identity. The four original species of the MTC are *M. tuberculosis* (affects humans, known as *M. tuberculosis sensu stricto*), *M. africanum* (affects humans), *M. microti* (affects voles) and *M. bovis* (affects cattle and other bovines). Newer species of the MTC include *M. pinnipedii* (affects pinnipeds: seals and sea lions), *M. canettii* (affects humans? it is the most ancestral recognized MTC member, although rarely isolated), the dassie bacillus (affects the rock hyraxes, [*Procavia capensis*]), *M. caprae* (affects goats), *Myco bacterium orygis*, (associated with various species), *Mycobacterium mungi* (which infects banded mongooses [*Mungos mungo*]), *Mycobacterium suricattae* (which affects meerkats [*Suricata suricattae*]), and *M. bovis*-BCG [1, 2]. The most accurate method to distinguish members of the MTC from one another are through genetic markers, single nucleotide polymorphisms (SNPs) in the 16S rDNA and gyrB genes and elsewhere in the genome, as well as extensive sequence polymorphisms referred to as regions of difference [2].

The deciphering of the *Mycobacterium tuberculosis* (MTB) genome that contains 4,411,529 base-pairs with high guanine-cytosine content [3] has allowed the reconstruction of the evolutionary history of MTB as an infectious agent at a global level. MTB emerged from Africa 70,000 years ago and followed human migrations and was forced to genetically evolve to be able to persist in these low-density migrant populations. The increase in human population density associated with the introduction of agriculture and overall civilization led to the selection and transmission of more virulent MTB strains, which are now known as modern MTB strains [4].

No human remains older than 11,000 years have shown the presence of tuberculosis disease, while the earliest tuberculosis case in animals has been reported in the 17,000-year-old remains of a bison [5].

Human disease by *M. bovis* strains is a frequent clinical finding, with transmission to the human host occurring via aerosol (in people in contact with livestock) or the consumption of infected milk. There has always been speculation that human TB originally was acquired as a zoonotic disease from cattle; the fact that animal tuberculosis preceded human tuberculosis suggests some causality with the increase in domestication of livestock. It has been hypothesized that contact of animal stocks and humans favored transmission from cattle to humans (in the past, humans shared their home with domesticated animals to protect them from the weather and predators). However, this hypothesis proved to be false when mycobacterial interspersed repetitive unit genotyping and whole-genome sequencing (WGS) provided strong evidence against such a linear explanation [5]; the accumulation of genomic deletions makes it improbable that *M. bovis* is the precursor of *M. tuberculosis* and that human TB was associated with the domestication of cattle [1].

Paleopathological studies had proven that mycobacterial disease was present in America in the pre-Columbian era [6] when *Mycobacterium tuberculosis* DNA was identified in a pre-Columbian Peruvian mummy [7]. It has been suggested that seals were the source of human tuberculosis in South America, predating the entrance of *Mycobacterium tuberculosis* L4 strains carried by the European Conquistadores. However, *M. pinnipedii* has been entirely replaced by the L4 lineage in the present day [8].

M. tuberculosis belongs to the order of the *Actinomycetales* and the *Myco bacteriaceae* family. It lacks capsule or flagella and does not produce spores or toxins; it stains very weakly as Gram-positive; it measures 0.5 by 4 μ. It is a preferably aerobic bacillus that, if necessary, can persist under anaerobic conditions. A distinctive feature of the *M. tuberculosis* cell wall is its content of N-glycolimuranic acid instead of N-acetylmuramic acid found in most bacteria. The unusual cell wall of *M. tuberculosis* allows it to survive inside the alveolar macrophage, a cell that usually destroys the bacteria that phagocytes.

Transmission of tuberculosis usually occurs through aerosols from one diseased host to a contact. Mycobacteria virulence will adapt to the host immunity. However, greater virulence would facilitate transmission, and it would also produce disseminated disease and some forms of TB that are nontransmissible (*e.g.*, TB meningitis), types of disease that would rapidly kill the host stopping the chain of transmission; therefore, excessive virulence could be detrimental to mycobacteria survival. Optimal transmissibility requires enough virulence to produce a disease with a high rate of transmission (*e.g.*, pulmonary disease through aerosols) before killing the host [1].

Mycobacterium tuberculosis is characterized by its slow growth rate (generation time in synthetic media is about 24 hours), dormancy (known clinically as latent TB infection), a sophisticated cell wall, and genetic homogeneity. The state of dormancy reflects metabolic shut down as a response to the cell-mediated immune response of the host, a response that will contain, but not sterilize the lesion. When immunity wanes (*e.g.*, old age) or the host immune response is inadequate (*e.g.*, due to immunosuppressive treatment or HIV co-infection), latent bacteria can reactivate, even decades after the primary infection [9].

One of the host responses to *M. tuberculosis* infection is the formation of a cluster of macrophages, creating a granuloma surrounding the mycobacteria. Host immune containment by granuloma formation creates a physical micro environment with nutrient limitations, a low pH, the presence of hydrolytic enzymes, and reduced oxygen tension. These granulomas are initially solid or caseous during latent infection, but when the immune pressure wanes (aging, immunosuppression by HIV infection, among others), the granuloma liquefies, allowing rapid bacterial replication and tissue damage. *M. tuberculosis* cultures with low oxygen tension (or anaerobic conditions) develop a thicker cell wall as an adaptation to low-oxygen conditions [10].

MTB cell wall (which stains weakly as a Gram-negative) constitutes a robust and highly impermeable barrier to harmful compounds and drugs. It includes an asymmetrical lipid bilayer made of mycolic acids on the inside and glycolipids and waxy components on the external layer. On the inside of the cell wall, there is a thin layer of peptidoglycan covalently linked to arabinogalactan and lipoarabinomannan, which in turn are bound to the mycolic acids. The mycolic acids retain the stain with carbol fuchsin or auramine when decolorized by acid alcohol, hence the term acid-fast bacilli. Two of the first-line antituberculosis drugs, isoniazid (mycolic acids), and ethambutol (arabinogalactan), target components of the cell wall.

MTB has several secretion systems, which are required for its full virulence. One of the secretion systems (ESX1) secretes among other antigens, ESAT-6 and CFP-10, antigens that are now used for the immunologic diagnosis of MTB infection in the interferon-gamma release assays (known as IGRA tests). *M. bovis*-BCG (an attenuated strain of wild *M. bovis*) has lost the ESX1 secretion system, and does not express ESAT-6 or CFP-10; therefore, IGRAs can be utilized to distinguish between *M. tuberculosis* infection and the immune reaction caused by BCG vaccination (unlike the tuberculin skin test).

MTB can sense when the local tissue conditions are inadequate for survival (low oxygen tension and nutrient depletion), as in the macrophages and granulomas, responding by the activation of a dormant state, in which the bacilli stop multiplying, down-regulates their metabolism and activate anaerobic metabolism. These dormant mycobacteria can persist in the host for years and revert to an active state when the conditions allow it (*e.g.*, immunosuppression) [4].

M. tuberculosis can synthesize all the essential amino acids, vitamins, and enzyme co-factors. It can also metabolize carbohydrates, hydrocarbons, alcohols, ketones, and carboxylic acids. Under aerobic conditions, adenosine triphosphate (ATP) will be generated by oxidative phosphorylation, but mycobacteria must adapt its metabolism to the microaerophilic and anaerobic environment present at the center of a granuloma.

M. tuberculosis is naturally resistant to many antibiotics. An essential factor in this resistance capacity is due mainly to its highly hydrophobic cell wall acting as a permeable physical barrier, but many resistance determinants are encoded in its genome, including hydrolases, β-lactamases and drug-efflux systems [9].

REFERENCES

[1]   Mostowy S, Behr MA. The origin and evolution of *Mycobacterium tuberculosis.* Clin Chest Med
       2005; 26(2): 207-216, v-vi.
       [http://dx.doi.org/10.1016/j.ccm.2005.02.004] [PMID: 15837106]

[2]   Clarke C, Van Helden P, Miller M, Parsons S. Animal-adapted members of the *Mycobacterium
       tuberculosis* complex endemic to the southern African subregion. J South African Vet Association
       2016; 87(1) a1322.
       [http://dx.doi.org/10.4102/ jsava. v87i1.1322]

[3]   Lin SY, Desmond EP. Molecular diagnosis of tuberculosis and drug resistance. Clin Lab Med 2014;
       34(2): 297-314.
       [http://dx.doi.org/10.1016/j.cll.2014.02.005] [PMID: 24856529]

[4]   Delogu G, Sali M, Fadda G. The biology of *mycobacterium tuberculosis* infection. Mediterr J Hematol
       Infect Dis 2013; 5(1): e2013070.
       [http://dx.doi.org/10.4084/mjhid.2013.070] [PMID: 24363885]

[5]   Rothschild BM, Martin LD, Lev G, *et al. Mycobacterium tuberculosis* complex DNA from an extinct
       bison dated 17,000 years before the present. Clin Infect Dis 2001; 33(3): 305-11.
       [http://dx.doi.org/10.1086/321886] [PMID: 11438894]

[6]   Stead WW, Eisenach KD, Cave MD, *et al.* When did *Mycobacterium tuberculosis* infection first occur
       in the New World? An important question with public health implications. Am J Respir Crit Care Med
       1995; 151(4): 1267-8.
       [http://dx.doi.org/10.1164/ajrccm.151.4.7697265] [PMID: 7697265]

[7]   Salo WL, Aufderheide AC, Buikstra J, Holcomb TA. Identification of *Mycobacterium tuberculosis*
       DNA in a pre-Columbian Peruvian mummy. Proc Natl Acad Sci USA 1994; 91(6): 2091-4.
       [http://dx.doi.org/10.1073/pnas.91.6.2091] [PMID: 8134354]

[8]   Barbier M, Wirth T. The evolutionary history, demography, and spread of the *Mycobacterium
       tuberculosis* complex. Microbiol Spectrum 2016; 4(4).
       [http://dx.doi.org/10.1128/microbiolspec.TBTB2-0008-2016]

[9]   Cole ST, Brosch R, Parkhill J, *et al.* Deciphering the biology of *Mycobacterium tuberculosis* from the
       complete genome sequence. Nature 1998; 393(6685): 537-44.
       [http://dx.doi.org/10.1038/31159] [PMID: 9634230]

[10]   Rosenkrands I, Slayden RA, Crawford J, Aagaard C, Barry CE III, Andersen P. Hypoxic response of
       mycobacterium tuberculosis studied by metabolic labeling and proteome analysis of cellular and
       extracellular proteins. J Bacteriol 2002; 184(13): 3485-91.
       [http://dx.doi.org/10.1128/JB.184.13.3485–3491.2002]

CHAPTER 3

Tuberculosis: A Natural History of the Disease

Abstract: Tuberculosis infection occurs when a subject inhales the *Mycobacterium tuberculosis* bacilli (MTB). An active case of pulmonary or laryngeal tuberculosis generates infectious particles called droplet nuclei of <5 microns in diameter, when coughing, sneezing or through any other forceful expiratory maneuver. The infectiousness of a patient with TB is directly related to the form of the disease (laryngeal, pulmonary), the presence of cough, cavitary lung disease and the positivity of the sputum smear/culture.

The prevalence of *M. tuberculosis* infection among household contacts is higher than 50%. Contacts who are <5 years of age or HIV infected have the most significant risk of developing tuberculosis once they acquire the infection.

In latent tuberculous infection, most bacilli are metabolically inactive, and only a few are replicating. In immunocompetent individuals, these bacilli are destroyed by the immune defenses of the host and the development of active disease aborts. When the immunity of the subject fails, the bacilli multiply, and eventually, active tuberculosis ensues. If latent infection tuberculosis is not treated, approximately 5% of infected individuals will develop the active disease within the first two years after infection, and another 5% will develop TB sometime later in life.

HIV infection is the most significant risk factor for the progression of LTBI to active TB disease, with an annual risk of 7-10% for subjects who are not receiving highly active antiretroviral treatment.

Keywords: Cavitary disease, Cough, Droplet nuclei, Immunity, Latent tuberculosis infection, T lymphocytes.

INTRODUCTION

Tuberculosis infection occurs when a subject inhales the *Mycobacterium tuberculosis* bacilli (MTB). Although there are other ways to acquire tuberculosis (ingestion of contaminated milk products, transdermal inoculation or transplacental) by far, the most common route is by inhalation.

An active case of pulmonary or laryngeal tuberculosis generates infectious particles called droplet nuclei of <5 microns in diameter when coughing, sneezing, shouting (or singing), or any other forceful expiratory maneuver;

depending on the environmental conditions, these particles can remain suspended in the air for several hours, and are inhaled by a susceptible individual who may become infected and develop active tuberculosis [1].

Four factors determine the probability of transmission of *M. tuberculosis*:

1. The susceptibility of the exposed individual that is directly related to the host immune status.
2. The infectiousness of the source case: the higher the number of bacilli expelled by the source case, the higher the degree of infectiousness.
3. The environmental conditions that affect the concentration of microorganisms.
4. The degree of exposure to the source case.

The infectivity of a patient with TB is directly related to the form of the disease (laryngeal, pulmonary), the presence of cough, cavitary lung disease, and the positivity of the sputum smear/culture.

Regarding the environmental conditions, the higher the concentration of *M. tuberculosis* in the air, the higher is the risk of transmission. Smaller, enclosed spaces with inadequate ventilation facilitate a higher concentration of droplet nuclei in the atmosphere, increasing the risk of infection.

Finally, the longer the duration and frequency of the exposure, and the closer the proximity to the source case, the higher the risk of transmission.

The highest probability of infection at home is when the index case is smear-positive, and the contact is less than 15 years old [2]. According to a recent systematic review and meta-analysis, the prevalence of *M. tuberculosis* infection among household contacts is higher than 50% [3]. Contacts who are <5 years of age or HIV infected have the most significant risk of developing active tuberculosis once they acquire the infection.

Due to its size (<5 microns), MTB traverse the mouth or nasal passages, upper respiratory tract, and bronchi to reach the alveoli, where it is then rapidly phagocytosed by the alveolar macrophages and contained in phagosomes. Other bacteria are usually destroyed when exposed to lysosome enzymes, but MTB has developed biological resistance mechanisms such as inhibition of phagosome-lysosome fusion and evading the lethal acid pH by staying within the phagolysosomes. In a tuberculosis-naïve individual that lacks specific immunity against tuberculosis, the macrophage is not able to kill MTB, and the bacilli actively replicate within it, protected from other immune cells. Therefore, alveolar macrophages initially constitute a niche for mycobacterial replication and serve as a reservoir for latent mycobacteria within pulmonary granulomas during latent tuberculosis infection (LTBI) [4].

Initially, due to the small number of bacilli, there is no specific immune response against MTB, allowing its replication and dissemination by hematogenous and lymphatic pathways to the rest of the body, including areas in which TB disease is most likely to develop: regional lymph nodes, apex of the lungs, suprarenal glands, kidneys, brain, and bones [5].

After 4-8 weeks in immunocompetent hosts, there is a specific immune response through a clone of T lymphocytes specifically sensitized to kill MTB. Neutrophils, lymphocytes and other immune cells migrate to the primary infection site to form a cellular infiltrate that will evolve, adopting the typical structure of a granuloma with macrophages, multinucleated cells and lipid-filled foamy macrophages surrounded by concentric circles of lymphocytes [6]. If the immune response is active, the granuloma will eventually calcify encapsulating the bacilli and protecting it from the host immune response; this primary lesion is known as the Ghon complex [7].

During latent infection, MTB is metabolically active and replicates in host tissues despite the lack of any clinical sign or symptom of the disease [8].

In latent tuberculous infection, most bacilli are metabolically inactive, and only a few are replicating. In immunocompetent individuals, these bacilli are destroyed by the immune defenses of the host, and the development of the active disease is aborted. When the immunity of the subject fails, the bacilli multiply actively, and eventually, active tuberculosis ensues [9, 10]. A classic example is the HIV infection that affects the CD4 T cells, which are essential for controlling the TB infection [11], treatment of rheumatic diseases with anti-TNF biologics [12], corticosteroid treatment, chronic renal disease [13], diabetes [14], cancer, hematological diseases [5], and other conditions that affect T cell function.

If latent infection tuberculosis is not treated, approximately 5% of infected individuals will develop the active disease within the first two years after infection, and another 5% will develop TB sometime later in life. Although everyone who has LTBI can develop active TB, some subjects are at higher risk. Due to the suppression of the cell-mediated immunity, HIV infection is the most significant risk factor for the progression of LTBI to active TB disease, with an annual risk of 7-10% for subjects who are not receiving highly active antiretroviral treatment; antiretroviral therapy reduces the risk of tuberculosis among people with HIV infection by 67% [15, 16]. For people with LTBI and diabetes, and with no adequate diabetes control, the risk is about 30% over a lifetime.

Untreated smear-positive tuberculosis among HIV negative individuals has a 10-year case fatality of 70%. The duration of disease from onset to cure or death is approximately three years and appears to be similar for smear-positive and smear-negative tuberculosis [17].

REFERENCES

[1]   Churchyard G, Kim P, Shah NS, *et al.* What we know about tuberculosis transmission: an overview. J Infect Dis 2017; 216(S6) (suppl_6): S629-35.
        [http://dx.doi.org/10.1093/infdis/jix362] [PMID: 29112747]

[2]   Zelner JL, Murray MB, Becerra MC, *et al.* Age-specific risks of tuberculosis infection from household and community exposures and opportunities for interventions in a high-burden setting. Am J Epidemiol 2014; 180(8): 853-61.
        [http://dx.doi.org/10.1093/aje/kwu192] [PMID: 25190676]

[3]   Fox GJ, Barry SE, Britton WJ, Marks GB. Contact investigation for tuberculosis: a systematic review and meta-analysis. Eur Respir J 2013; 41(1): 140-56.
        [http://dx.doi.org/10.1183/09031936.00070812] [PMID: 22936710]

[4]   Sia JK, Georgieva M, Rengarajan J. innate immune defenses in human tuberculosis: an overview of the interactions between *mycobacterium tuberculosis* and innate immune cells. J Immunol Res 2015; 2015: 747543.
        [http://dx.doi.org/10.1155/2015/747543] [PMID: 26258152]

[5]   Delogu G, Sali M, Fadda G. The biology of *mycobacterium tuberculosis* infection. Mediterr J Hematol Infect Dis 2013; 5(1): e2013070.
        [http://dx.doi.org/10.4084/mjhid.2013.070] [PMID: 24363885]

[6]   Saunders BM, Cooper AM. Restraining mycobacteria: role of granulomas in mycobacterial infections. Immunol Cell Biol 2000; 78(4): 334-41.
        [http://dx.doi.org/10.1046/j.1440-1711.2000.00933.x] [PMID: 10947857]

[7]   Ghon N. The primary complex in human tuberculosis and its significance. Am Rev Tuberc 1923; 7(5): 314-7.

[8]   Gideon HP, Flynn JL. Latent tuberculosis: what the host "sees"? Immunol Res 2011; 50(2-3): 202-12.
        [http://dx.doi.org/10.1007/s12026-011-8229-7] [PMID: 21717066]

[9]   Chao MC, Rubin EJ. Letting sleeping dos lie: does dormancy play a role in tuberculosis? Annu Rev Microbiol 2010; 64: 293-311.
        [http://dx.doi.org/10.1146/annurev.micro.112408.134043] [PMID: 20825351]

[10]   Gengenbacher M, Kaufmann SHE. *Mycobacterium tuberculosis*: success through dormancy. FEMS Microbiol Rev 2012; 36(3): 514-32.
        [http://dx.doi.org/10.1111/j.1574-6976.2012.00331.x] [PMID: 22320122]

[11]   Pawlowski A, Jansson M, Sköld M, Rottenberg ME, Källenius G. Tuberculosis and HIV co-infection. PLoS Pathog 2012; 8(2): e1002464.
        [http://dx.doi.org/10.1371/journal.ppat.1002464] [PMID: 22363214]

[12]   Bruns H, Meinken C, Schauenberg P, *et al.* Anti-TNF immunotherapy reduces CD8+ T cell-mediated antimicrobial activity against *Mycobacterium tuberculosis* in humans. J Clin Invest 2009; 119(5): 1167-77.
        [http://dx.doi.org/10.1172/JCI38482] [PMID: 19381021]

[13]   Bedi RS. Management of tuberculosis in special situations. Lung India 2005; 22: 138-41.

[14]   Lin Y, Harries AD, Kumar AMV, *et al.* Management of diabetes mellitus-tuberculosis: a guide to the essential practice. Paris, France: International Union Against Tuberculosis and Lung Disease 2019.

[15] Lawn SD, Wood R, De Cock KM, Kranzer K, Lewis JJ, Churchyard GJ. Antiretrovirals and isoniazid preventive therapy in the prevention of HIV-associated tuberculosis in settings with limited health-care resources. Lancet Infect Dis 2010; 10(7): 489-98.
[http://dx.doi.org/10.1016/S1473-3099(10)70078-5] [PMID: 20610331]

[16] Zachariah R, Bemelmans M, Akesson A, *et al.* Reduced tuberculosis case notification associated with scaling up antiretroviral treatment in rural Malawi. Int J Tuberc Lung Dis 2011; 15(7): 933-7.
[http://dx.doi.org/10.5588/ijtld.10.0666] [PMID: 21682967]

[17] Tiemersma EW, van der Werf MJ, Borgdorff MW, Williams BG, Nagelkerke NJD. Natural history of tuberculosis: duration and fatality of untreated pulmonary tuberculosis in HIV negative patients: a systematic review. PLoS One 2011; 6(4): e17601.
[http://dx.doi.org/10.1371/journal.pone.0017601] [PMID: 21483732]

CHAPTER 4

Clinical Diagnosis of Tuberculosis

Abstract: Symptoms and signs of active tuberculosis (TB) depend on its anatomical location. Pulmonary disease is the most common presentation of tuberculosis in the adult patient (more than 80% of the cases in the immunocompetent patient). Signs and symptoms can appear after just a few weeks from the primary infection, or many years later due to the reactivation of latent disease anywhere in the body.

Symptoms of pulmonary tuberculosis are nonspecific and may occur in many other pulmonary conditions; however, in high-burden regions, they remain a valuable tool for initial screening.

Signs and symptoms of extrapulmonary tuberculosis (EPTB) are protean, and chest x-rays of the chest frequently do not show abnormalities. TB lymphadenitis is the most common form of EPTB, especially in children and young individuals.

Miliary tuberculosis is characterized by the presence of disseminated innumerable small nodules. It is secondary to the hematogenous spread of the bacilli throughout the body after the primary infection or the reactivation of a latent focus.

Although TB can involve any segment of the gastrointestinal tract, the ileocecal region is the most frequently affected. It is due to the ingestion of milk or milk products contaminated with *M. bovis*, the swallowing of secretions infected with *M. tuberculosis*, hematogenous dissemination of active TB disease, or from direct spread from contiguous organs.

Central nervous system tuberculosis is a consequence of hematogenous dissemination and the most severe form of the disease, with high morbimortality.

Keywords: Extrapulmonary, Lymphadenitis, Meningeal, Osteomyelitis, Pulmonary, Pericardial, Renal, Tuberculosis.

INTRODUCTION

Pulmonary Tuberculosis

Symptoms and signs of active tuberculosis depend on its anatomical location. Pulmonary disease is the most common presentation of tuberculosis in the adult patient (more than 80% of the cases in the immunocompetent patient), although the condition can appear at any age. It is also the second most contagious form of TB and the primary source of transmission among human populations.

Signs and symptoms can appear from just a few weeks from the primary infection to many years later due to the reactivation of latent disease anywhere in the body. Most patients are male (2:1 male to female ratio).

Reactivation TB is a progressive disease (very seldom self-limited). Sometimes is rapidly fatal (in severely immunosuppressed hosts), but most cases have a prolonged subclinical stage (2-3 months).

Symptoms of pulmonary tuberculosis are nonspecific and may occur in many other pulmonary conditions; however, in high-burden regions, they remain a valuable tool for initial screening, and in case of clinical suspicion to carry out the confirmatory laboratory studies.

Pulmonary TB may cause the following symptoms: cough (initially non-productive) that lasts ≥3 weeks, production of sputum, usually purulent, dyspnea, hemoptoic sputum or frank hemoptysis and chest pain. Constitutional symptoms include fatigue (can be present for weeks, before the other symptoms appear), fever, chills, diaphoresis, anorexia, and inexplicable weight loss. If there is pleural involvement, pleuritic pain will occur, usually dull, and subacute. The accumulation of fluid in the pleural cavity will separate the parietal from the visceral pleural layer, and the pain may disappear (despite the persistence of pleural inflammation and pleural fluid).

These symptoms are usually insidious, appearing progressively over the course of weeks, mistaken frequently for recurrent bouts of upper respiratory tract infection or community-acquired pneumonia that has not responded to conventional antibiotic therapy.

Chronic cases can develop dysphonia due to TB laryngitis, and swallowing of infected secretions can lead to gastrointestinal disease (TB enteritis, anorectal abscesses, and fistulas).

In some cases, asthenia can be severe due to hyponatremia caused by inappropriate secretion of antidiuretic hormone syndrome.

A small percentage of the patients with early active disease might not have any signs or symptoms and will be discovered during contact investigation due to an abnormal chest radiograph taken as part of the diagnostic protocol.

It is essential to investigate subjects exposed to a known case of tuberculosis in the family, friends, or at work. In the case of positive history, inquiries must be made about the possible index case regarding drug susceptibility, adherence to treatment, *etc*.

On physical examination, the patient might be febrile and look cachectic due to weight loss. Clinical signs during chest examination, besides those of a pleural effusion, are seldom useful for diagnosis, even though the patient might present extensive lesions on the chest radiography. In chronic cases, tracheal retraction due to fibrotic retraction of the upper lobes can be detected during neck examination.

The prognosis for pulmonary TB (especially for patients with pan-sensitive MTB strains) is usually good (cure rate >90%), if the patient completes his/her treatment [1].

Extrapulmonary Tuberculosis (EPTB)

Extrapulmonary TB (EPTB) is the result of the hematogenous and lymphatic dissemination of *M. tuberculosis* bacilli. Although dissemination usually happens during the primary infection, it is controlled by the immune system in more than 90% of immunocompetent individuals. The host immune response leads to the formation of encapsulated granulomas, which contain viable mycobacteria in a latent stage. However, alterations in the cell-mediated immune response mechanisms like extreme ages, immunosuppression due to coexisting medical conditions (HIV co-infection, diabetes or chronic renal disease) or immunosuppressant treatment predispose to the reactivation of latent TB and the development of the active disease.

Signs and symptoms are protean, and chest x-rays frequently do not show abnormalities. The diagnosis requires a high index of suspicion, and delays in the diagnosis are frequent with the consequent increase in morbimortality.

As EPTB is a systemic disease, the simultaneous involvement of several organs and systems is not infrequent, detection of which will depend on the accuracy of the diagnostic protocol.

The definitive diagnosis of EPTB requires obtaining fluids or tissues through fine-needle or open biopsy for molecular testing (Xpert MTB/RIF) and mycobacterial culture [2].

Pleural Tuberculosis

Pleural tuberculosis is the second most common form of extrapulmonary TB (EPTB). The frequency of pleural TB varies according to endemicity (low burden areas 3-5%, *vs*. up to 30% in regions with a high burden of disease) [3].

As with pulmonary TB, pleural TB can present as either primary or reactivation disease. Symptoms typically include fever, chills, dyspnea, weight loss, and pleuritic chest pain (usually dull, and subacute); the accumulation of fluid in the pleural cavity separates the parietal from the visceral pleural layer, and the pain may disappear (despite the persistence of pleural inflammation). The effusion is self-limited, resolving without treatment; however, if not treated, two-thirds of the patients progress to pulmonary TB within 5 years. TB pleural effusions are more frequent in patients co-infected with HIV; these patients also have a higher incidence of disseminated disease in comparison with non-HIV patients, with a more variegated clinical presentation, including high fever, diaphoresis, asthenia, diarrhea, hepatosplenomegaly and lymphadenopathy [1, 4].

Pleural fluid in TB is a straw-colored exudate, with high levels of lactic dehydro genase (more than 60% than that of the serum) and proteins (more than 50% than that of the serum); white cells predominance depends on the chronicity of the effusion; initially, there is a preponderance of neutrophils; later, the effusion has lymphocytes almost exclusively; glucose levels in the pleural fluid are low compared to that of the serum.

Adenosine deaminase (ADA) is an enzyme found in T-lymphocytes; the enzyme has two isoforms, ADA1 and ADA2; the latter is the predominant isoform in TB pleural effusions.

This test has been extensively used in high burden regions, where an ADA value of >40 IU/L combined with a lymphocytic effusion has a positive predictive value of 98%.

ADA levels can give false-positive results in rheumatoid pleural effusions, bacterial pleural infection, mesothelioma, lung cancer, and hematological malignancies, especially lymphoma.

The definitive diagnosis of TB pleural effusion consists of the demonstration of MTB bacilli in sputum, pleural fluid, or pleural biopsy specimens.

Tuberculosis Empyema

It can be the consequence of direct spread from pulmonary TB or a rupture lymph node. An exudative phase is followed by a fibrinopurulent phase, in which the purulent fluid is rich in microorganisms; if not treated adequately, it progresses to pleural fibrosis and lung entrapment that eventually calcifies. Occasionally the empyema drains directly into the thoracic surface (empyema necessitans) or provokes a bronchopleural fistula. A fibrothorax (pleural thickening and fibrotic retraction) occurs in up to 50% of the cases of empyema if not treated, with the consequent lung function impairment and dyspnea [3].

Miliary Tuberculosis

Miliary tuberculosis is characterized by the presence of disseminated, innumerable small nodules (millet seeds-like that correspond to tissue granulomas) detected in a chest x-ray. It is secondary to the hematogenous spread of the bacilli throughout the body after the primary infection or the reactivation of a latent focus. As mentioned, it is a form of disease of immunocompromised individuals (*e.g.*, the elderly, HIV infected individuals, chronic renal disease, solid organ transplant recipients, anti-TNF therapy, *etc.*). Although it can affect any organ, the most frequently affected are the lung, the liver, the spleen, the meninges, the bone marrow, and the adrenal glands. Most cases have a subacute presentation with insidious symptoms, but occasionally presentation is acute and severe, with septic shock and acute respiratory distress syndrome. It is diagnosed when the chest x-rays show the typical micronodular infiltrates; clinical manifestations may precede these radiographic findings for up to 2 or 3 weeks, but due to its higher sensitivity, they can be detected earlier with a chest CT scan, not only in the lung but also in the liver and spleen. During the physical examination, one can find choroidal tubercles in the ocular fundus that are associated with meningeal tuberculosis [1, 2].

TB Lymphadenitis

It is the most common form of EPTB, especially in children and young adults. It accounts for a third of all EPTB cases. The most common location is cervical lymphadenitis, although it can affect virtually all lymphatic chains. Frequently involves the cervical and supraclavicular chains, with lymph nodes that often coalesce, are hard to the touch, and painless. Later, they can present necrosis, fluctuate, and ulcerate with fistula formation; this form of lymphadenitis was known as scrofula [1, 2].

Mediastinal lymphadenitis is usually secondary to pulmonary disease, and their swelling can compress the trachea or esophagus.

Diagnosis in accessible lymph nodes can be obtained through fine-needle aspiration biopsy (FNAB), guided with ultrasound if necessary, for microbiological and molecular tests. A surgical biopsy is only needed if the fine needle aspiration biopsy FNAB has not been diagnostic [5].

Osteoarticular Tuberculosis

Tuberculosis can affect any bone or joint, but 50% of the cases of osteoarticular

TB affect the spine. Spondylitis (known as Pott disease) starts as an inflammation of the anterior aspect of the vertebral body, spreading to the intervertebral disk and adjacent vertebrae. In advanced cases, the infection spreads to the paravertebral soft tissues with the formation of abscesses, finally affecting the posterior region of the vertebral body and involving the spinal cord. Pott's disease mainly affects the thoracolumbar area of the spine. Back pain is the most common symptom. Paraplegia in spinal TB has several stages, from negligible weakness after walking in the early stages to complete paraplegia in advanced stages. Radiographic studies (simple x-rays or CT scans) are needed to determine the extension of the disease. Magnetic Resonance Imaging (MRI) is the study of choice to assess possible neurological involvement [2]. Definitive diagnosis requires CT guided biopsy to obtain tissue for microbiologic, molecular, and histopathological studies [6].

Gastrointestinal Tuberculosis

Although TB can involve any segment of the gastrointestinal tract (GI-TB), the ileocecal region is the most frequently affected, followed by the colon and small intestine; the esophagus and stomach are rarely involved. GI-TB is associated with the ingestion of milk or milk products contaminated with *M. bovis*, the swallowing of secretions infected with *M. tuberculosis*, hematogenous dissemination of active TB disease, or from direct spread from contiguous organs. Signs and symptoms, as with other types of EPTB, are nonspecific: abdominal pain, a palpable abdominal mass, anorexia, fever, diaphoresis, weight loss, diarrhea (or constipation), hematochezia, fistulas, and intestinal strictures. The latter leads to bowel obstruction, a common complication of GI-TB. Definite diagnosis depends on the identification of *M. tuberculosis* complex in biopsy material obtained through colonoscopy.

Peritoneal tuberculosis is usually a consequence of hematogenous spread (or the spread from GI-TB or genitourinary TB), especially in patients with immunosuppression (HIV infection, diabetes) and in patients undergoing peritoneal dialysis. Complications of peritoneal TB include the accumulation of ascites fluid, an exudate like that of pleural TB; some patients develop peritoneal adhesions. Acid-fast bacilli (AFB) smears of peritoneal fluid have very low sensitivity (less than 5%), while the culture of the ascites fluid has a yield reported as high as 80%. In cases where the analysis of the ascites fluid is nondiagnostic, a laparoscopic biopsy will be required [1, 2, 7].

Central Nervous System Tuberculosis (CNS-TB)

CNS-TB is a consequence of hematogenous dissemination and the most severe form of the disease, with high morbimortality. The disease can manifest itself as a cerebral tuberculoma, periarteritis with vascular obstruction and ischemic stroke, arachnoiditis (and obstructive hydrocephalus) and meningitis, the most common presentation.

TB meningitis is a subacute disease with a spectrum that goes from headaches to progressive lethargy, coma, and death in most untreated patients. In the early stages, patients are febrile but without neurologic compromise, while in advanced stages, patients have severe sensorium deterioration and hemiparesis or hemiplegia. It mainly affects the basal meninges with the involvement of cranial nerves (III, IV, and VI) and oculomotor dysfunction. MRI is considered the gold standard for diagnosis. Cerebral spinal fluid (CSF) in patients with meningitis shows a high concentration of proteins and low glucose with monocyte pleocytosis. Phenotypic diagnosis (smears and culture) have a low yield. The Xpert MTB/RIF offers now the opportunity to quickly establish the diagnosis (less than 2 hours) with an acceptable sensitivity (79.5%) and excellent specificity (98.6%) *vs.* the culture as the gold standard [2, 8, 9].

Genitourinary TB (GU-TB)

GU-TB is a consequence of hematogenous dissemination during primary or miliary TB [10, 11]. Initially, GU-TB is asymptomatic, but with the involvement of the bladder, symptoms suggestive of lower urinary tract infection are common; urinalysis reveals sterile pyuria and microscopic hematuria, and in later stages, the ureteral stricture can lead to urinary obstruction and hydronephrosis. Imaging studies (ultrasound, pyelograms, and CT scans) are useful auxiliary tests, although the definite diagnosis requires the identification of *M. tuberculosis* by culture. Molecular testing (Xpert MTB/RIF) has very high sensitivity (95% *versus* culture as the gold standard) [12].

Tuberculosis can also affect the reproductive system causing prostatitis, epididymitis, and orchitis in males and bilateral involvement of the Fallopian tubes in females; it is a common cause of infertility in developing countries. Diagnosis requires the identification of *M. tuberculosis* in prostate fluid or tissue biopsy, menstrual fluid, or endometrial biopsy [12].

Laryngeal Tuberculosis

Laryngeal tuberculosis is a complication of pulmonary disease, with the involvement of the laryngeal structures and the development of ulcers and nodules in the vocal cords. The most common symptoms are dysphonia, cough, and stridor. It is considered the most infectious form of tuberculosis [13].

Tuberculosis Pericarditis

It can be a consequence of direct spread from adjacent organs or structures (lung, lymph nodes, esophagus, spine, *etc.*) or of hematogenous dissemination. Pericardial tuberculosis is rarely a localized disease. Echocardiography is the imaging study of choice to detect pericardial effusion and complications such as constrictive pericarditis and cardiac tamponade. As with pleural and peritoneal fluid, pericardial effusion is a monocytic exudate. The sensitivity of microbiologic studies (smears and cultures) is low, and thoracoscopic pericardial biopsy for bacteriologic and histopathologic studies is necessary to establish the diagnosis [1, 2, 14].

REFERENCES

[1]   Farga V, Caminero JA. Tuberculosis. Tercera Edición, Editorial Mediterráneo. Capítulo 2011; 6: 101-8.

[2]   Ramírez-Lapausa M, Menéndez-Saldaña A, Noguerado-Asensio A. Extrapulmonary tuberculosis: an overview. Rev Esp Sanid Penit 2015; 17(1): 3-11.
[http://dx.doi.org/10.4321/S1575-06202015000100002] [PMID: 25803112]

[3]   Shaw JA, Irusen EM, Diacon AH, Koegelenberg CF. Pleural tuberculosis: A concise clinical review. Clin Respir J 2018; 12(5): 1779-86.
[http://dx.doi.org/10.1111/crj.12900] [PMID: 29660258]

[4]   Gopi A, Madhavan SM, Sharma SK, Sahn SA. Diagnosis and treatment of tuberculous pleural effusion in 2006. Chest 2007; 131(3): 880-9.
[http://dx.doi.org/10.1378/chest.06-2063] [PMID: 17356108]

[5]   Lewinsohn DM, Leonard MK, LoBue PA, *et al.* Official American Thoracic Society/Infectious Diseases Society of America/Centers for Disease Control and Prevention Clinical Practice Guidelines: Diagnosis of Tuberculosis in Adults and Children. Clin Infect Dis 2017; 64(2): e1-e33.
[http://dx.doi.org/10.1093/cid/ciw694] [PMID: 27932390]

[6]   Kumar K. Spinal tuberculosis, natural history of disease, classifications and principles of management with historical perspective. Eur J Orthop Surg Traumatol 2016; 26(6): 551-8.
[http://dx.doi.org/10.1007/s00590-016-1811-x] [PMID: 27435619]

[7]   Choi EH, Coyle WJ. Gastrointestinal tuberculosis. Microbiol Spectrum 2016; 4(6): 0014.
[http://dx.doi.org/10.1128/microbiolspec.TNMI7-0014-2016]

[8]   World Health Organization. World Health Organization 2013. Automated real-time nucleic acid amplification technology for rapid and simultaneous detection of tuberculosis and rifampicin resistance: Xpert MTB/RIF assay for the diagnosis of pulmonary and extrapulmonary TB in adults and children. Policy update. World Health Organization. WHO/HTM/TB/201316 ISBN: 978 92 4 150633 5 2013.

[9]   Espinosa-Gimeno A, Martínez-Sanz J, Asong-Engonga L, Rodríguez-Zapata M. Protocolo diagnóstico y terapéutico de las tuberculosis extrapulmonares. Medicine (Baltimore) 2014; 11(52): 3091-7.

[10]   Figueiredo AA, Lucon AM. Urogenital tuberculosis: update and review of 8961 cases from the world literature. Rev Urol 2008; 10(3): 207-17.
[PMID: 18836557]

[11]   Figueiredo AA, Lucon AM, Srougi M. Urogenital tuberculosis. Microbiol Spectr 2017; 5(1)
[http://dx.doi.org/10.1128/microbiolspec.TNMI7-0015-2016] [PMID: 28087922]

[12]   Pang Y, Shang Y, Lu J, *et al.* GeneXpert MTB/RIF assay in the diagnosis of urinary tuberculosis from urine specimens. Sci Rep 2017; 7(1): 6181.
[http://dx.doi.org/10.1038/s41598-017-06517-0] [PMID: 28733605]

[13]   Yencha MW, Linfesty R, Blackmon A. Laryngeal tuberculosis. Am J Otolaryngol 2000; 21(2): 122-6.
[http://dx.doi.org/10.1016/S0196-0709(00)85010-3] [PMID: 10758999]

[14]   Chang SA. Tuberculous and infectious pericarditis. Cardiol Clin 2017; 35(4): 615-22.
[http://dx.doi.org/10.1016/j.ccl.2017.07.013] [PMID: 29025551]

CHAPTER 5

Imaging in Tuberculosis

Abstract: Tuberculosis is an excellent simulator and can mimic virtually any disease. Clinically, it has been divided into primary and post-primary tuberculosis. Primary tuberculosis usually refers to patients not previously exposed to *M. tuberculosis*. Primary tuberculosis is more frequent in children, with its highest prevalence in children under five years, although the frequency of primary forms in adults is increasing. The primary disease has four main presentations at imaging: chest lymphadenopathy, pneumonia, miliary disease, and pleural effusion. Post-primary TB (also known as reactivation or secondary TB) most commonly involves the lungs in the apical and posterior segments of the upper lobes and the apical segment of the lower lobes. Initially, there are parenchymal consolidations, that if they are not diagnosed and treated, usually progress to necrosis and cavitation. Unilateral lung destruction is a serious complication of pulmonary TB that occurs in chronic advanced cases. Although TB is mostly limited to the lungs, it can happen in any other tissue or organ, especially in the immunocompromised host.

Keywords: Atelectasis, Cavitation, Fibrosis, Lymphadenopathy, Miliary, Pleural effusion, Pneumonia, Tuberculosis.

INTRODUCTION

Tuberculosis (TB) is an excellent simulator and can mimic virtually any disease. Chest radiographs are still the primary imaging method, but computed tomography (CT) and magnetic resonance imaging (MRI) may be helpful in the evaluation of pulmonary and extrapulmonary disease [1].

PRIMARY TUBERCULOSIS

This term usually refers to patients not previously exposed to *M. tuberculosis*. It is more frequent in children, with its highest prevalence in children under five years, although the frequency of primary forms in adults is increasing. It is important to emphasize that chest radiographs can be normal in up to 15% of patients with proven pulmonary TB [2].

The primary disease has four main presentations at imaging: chest lymphadenopathy, pneumonia, miliary disease, and pleural effusion [3].

Rafael Laniado-Laborín

Chest lymphadenopathy is a frequent finding in children (almost in 100% of the cases), but nearly 50% of adults also present with this finding. It is usually unilaterally located in the hilum and right paratracheal region (Fig. **1**).

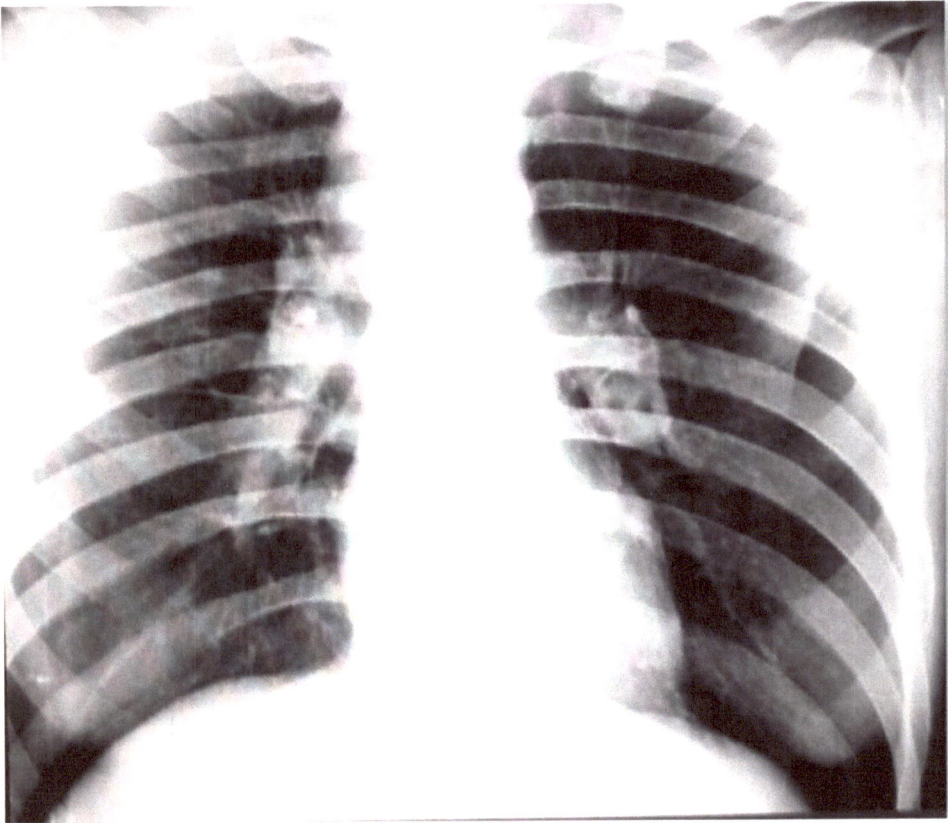

Fig. (1). Bilateral hilar and paratracheal adenopathy without apparent parenchymal involvement.

Lymphadenopathy is typically associated with other radiographic findings (parenchymal involvement), but it may be the only radiographic finding. CT has higher sensitivity to detect nodal disease, and frequently, larger nodes (>2 cm in diameter) may show a low attenuation center due to necrosis.

Parenchymal findings in primary TB are characterized by dense airspace disease, predominantly in the middle and lower lobes. It is indistinguishable by imaging from bacterial community-acquired pneumonia, although lymphadenopathy, if present, suggests a chronic etiology (tuberculosis or fungal pneumonia); also, the lack of response to conventional antibiotics should indicate the probability of *M. tuberculosis* as an etiologic agent (Fig. **2**).

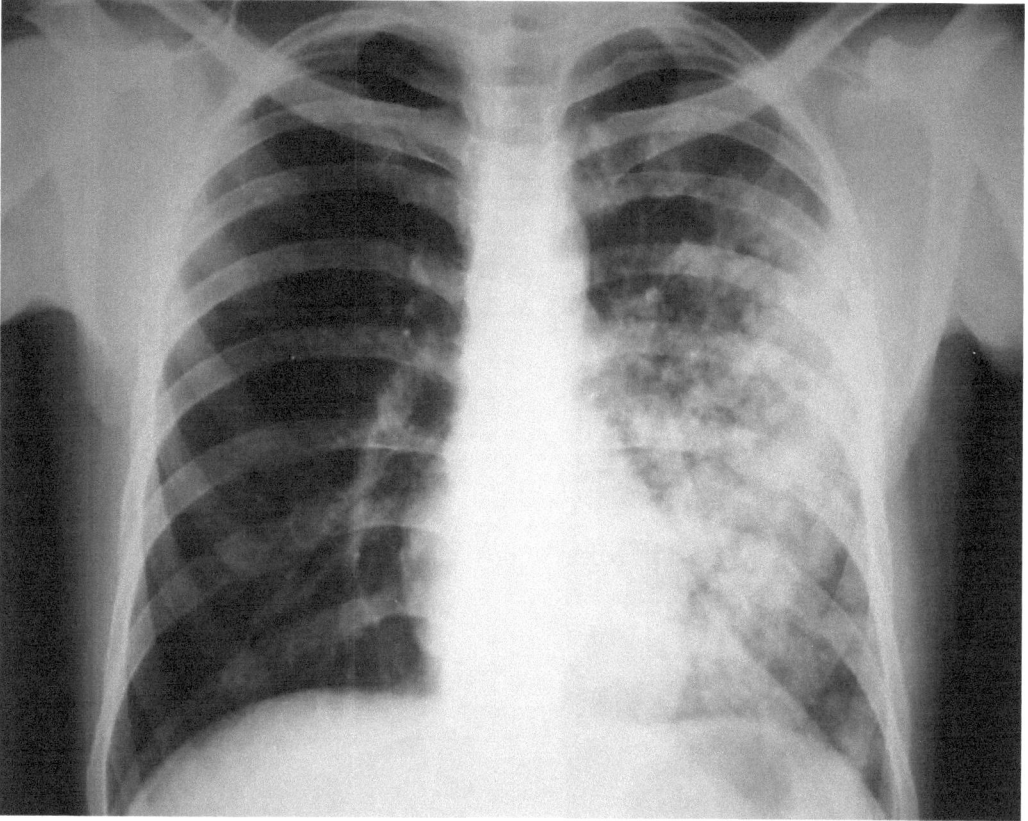

Fig. (2). TB pneumonia of the left upper lobe, including the lingula.

In most cases, TB pneumonia resolves without sequelae; occasionally, a calcified scar is evident in the chest radiograph, known as a Ghon focus. The combination of the Ghon focus and calcified hilar nodes (known as Ranke complex) is suggestive of TB, although it can also result from fungal disease (*e.g.*, coccidioidomycosis or histoplasmosis).

Miliary TB is secondary to the lymphohematogenous widespread dissemination of *M. tuberculosis*, frequently affecting highly vascularized organs (liver, lungs, spleen, bone marrow, kidneys, and suprarenal glands). Miliary disease is seen mainly at the extremes of age and in the immunocompromised patient. Initially, chest radiographs may be normal, and the typical findings evolve as the disease progresses. High-resolution CT is the imaging method of choice due to its higher sensitivity, and it can demonstrate the miliary pattern before the chest radiograph does [4].

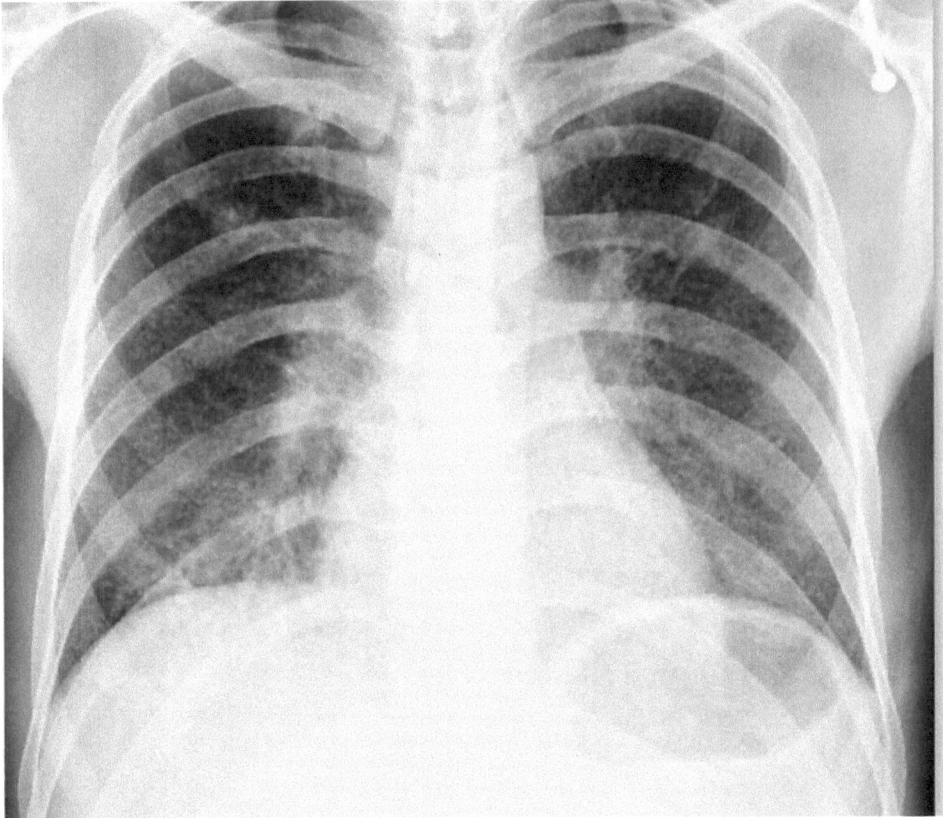

Fig. (3). Miliary tuberculosis. Disseminated lung nodules randomly distributed in the lung.

The characteristic findings consist of innumerable nodules, 1-3 mm in diameter, randomly distributed in the lungs (Fig. **3**). With effective antituberculosis treatment, the nodules usually resolve within 6 months without sequelae.

Frequently, the patients have additional radiographic abnormalities besides the miliary pattern (cavitation, pleural effusions, and lymphadenopathies).

Tuberculous pleural effusion can be a manifestation of primary or reactivation TB. It can be the only radiographic anomaly or be associated with lung parenchymal disease. It is radiographically indistinguishable from effusions from other etiologies (Figs. **4** and **5**).

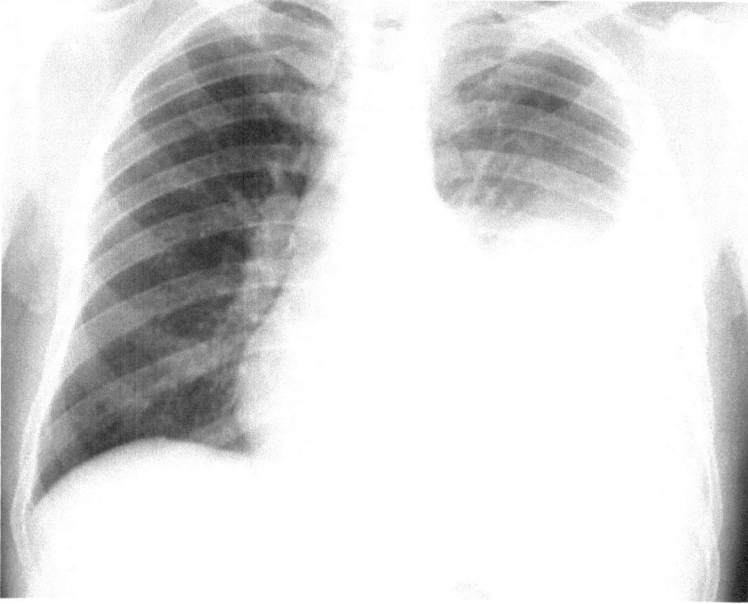

Fig. (4). Left pleural effusion as a manifestation of primary TB, with homogeneous opacity with a concave upper limit.

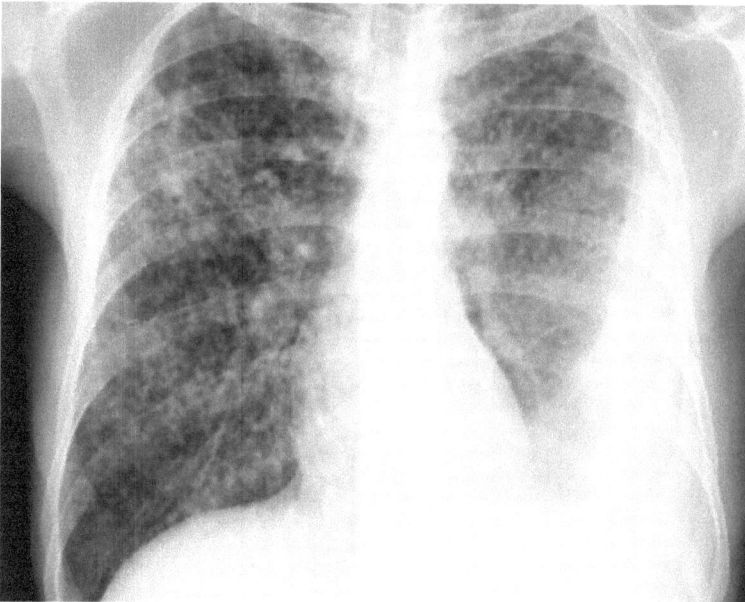

Fig. (5). Left pleural effusion with disseminated airspace opacities in a patient with TB and HIV co-infection.

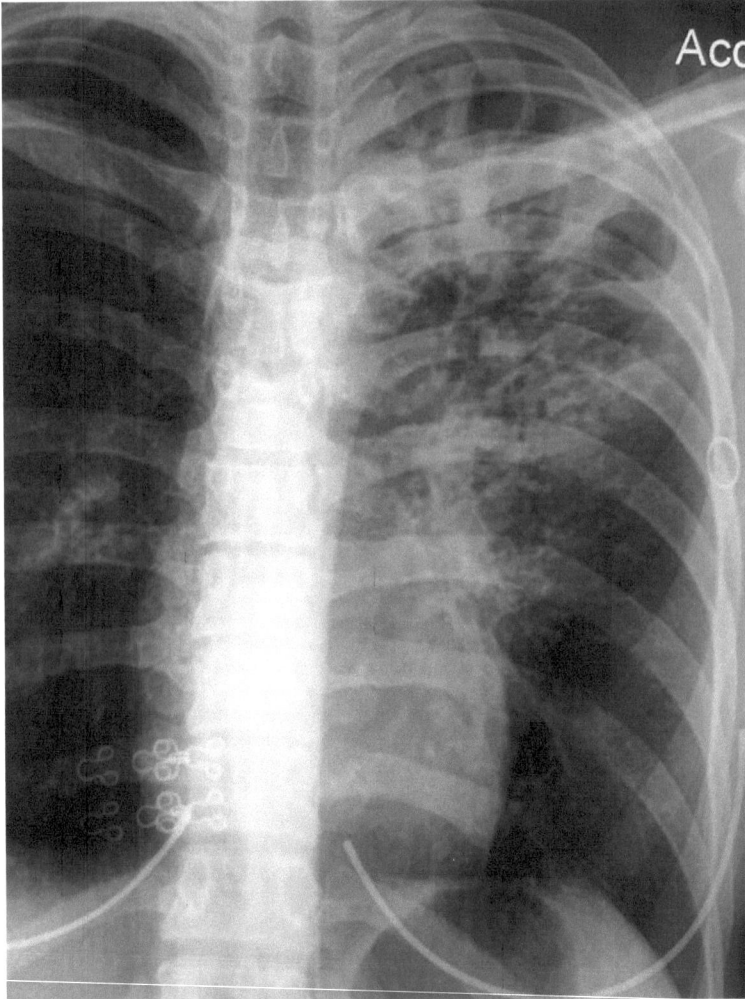

Fig. (6). Post-primary TB. Left upper lobe pneumonia with multiple cavities with air-fluid levels.

REACTIVATION (POST-PRIMARY) TUBERCULOSIS

Post-primary TB (also known as reactivation or secondary TB) most commonly involves the lungs, the apical and posterior segments of the upper lobes and the apical segment of the lower lobes. Initially, there are parenchymal consolidations, which, if not diagnosed and treated, usually progress to necrosis and cavitation (Fig. **6**). Air-fluid levels have been reported to occur occasionally in tuberculous cavities.

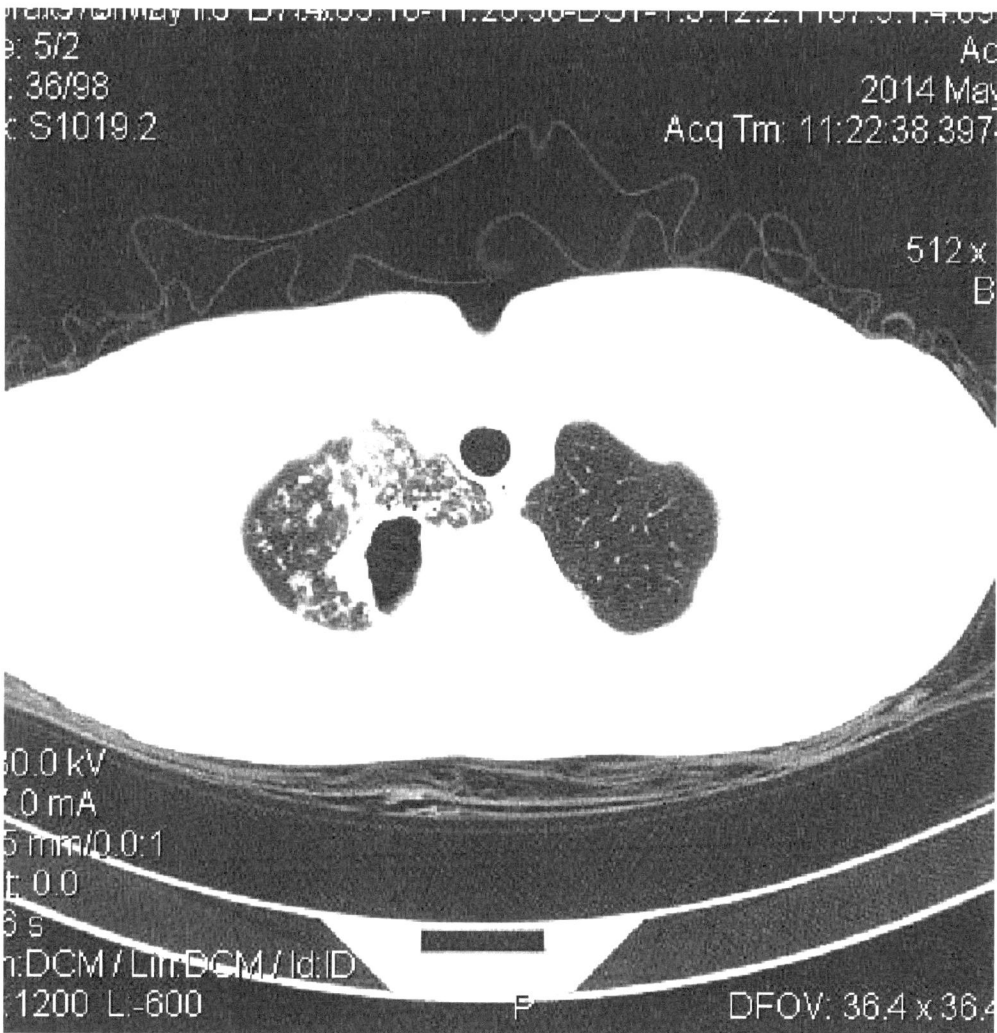

Fig. (7). Thick-walled cavity in the right upper lobe and airspace opacities surrounding it (CT scan).

The walls of the cavities can range from thin and smooth to thick and irregular (Fig. 7) [5].

In addition to these typical findings, due to bronchogenic spread, there are usually airspace and nodular opacities in other areas of the lungs, including the contralateral lung. Endobronchial spread occurs when necrotic lesion liquefies and drains into the bronchial tree [1].

If the patient receives effective antituberculosis treatment, lung cavities can disappear; thin-walled cavities usually collapse, leaving a fibrous scar; sometimes, they remain as air-filled cysts. Thick-walled cavities often persist as sequelae even after attaining bacteriologically cure.

Unlike the initial presentation of TB, hilar or mediastinal lymphadenopathy are uncommon in post-primary TB. Nodes greater than 2 cm in diameter that show a low attenuation center due to necrosis in a CT scan are highly suggestive of active disease (Fig. **8**).

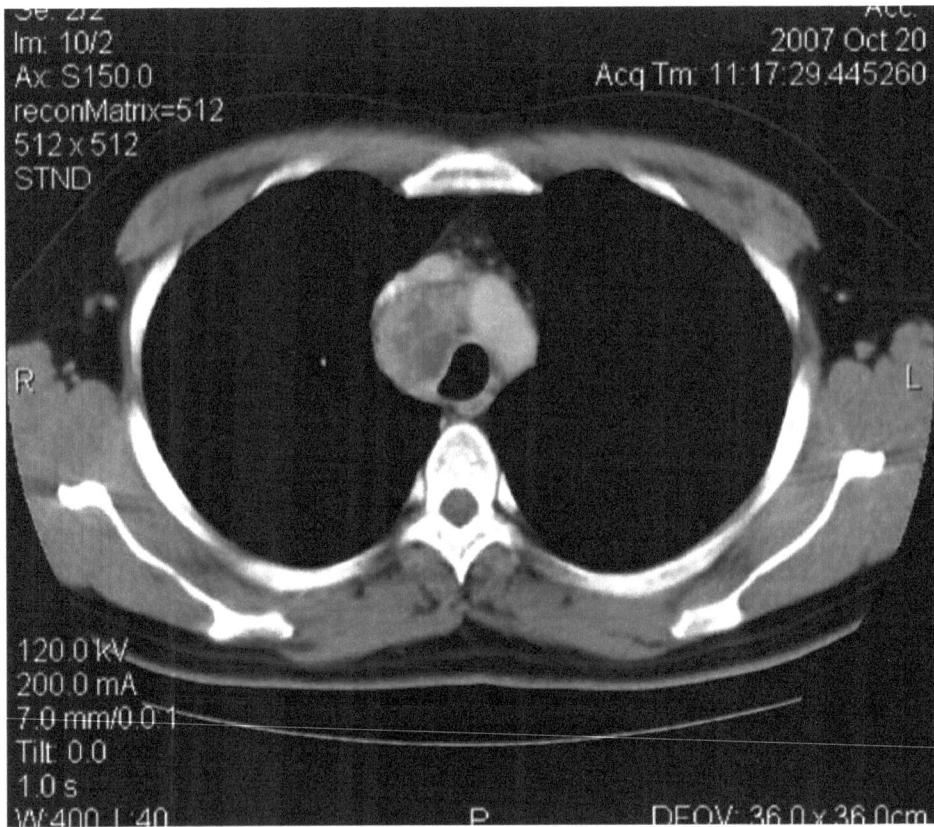

Fig. (8). Mediastinal adenopathy with low attenuation center that compresses the trachea.

Unilateral lung destruction is a serious complication of pulmonary TB that occurs in chronic advanced cases. It is frequently associated with bronchiectasis, that are easily colonized by bacteria (*e.g. Pseudomonas* spp.) and fungi that contribute to morbidity and mortality. Chest x-rays show a heterogeneous opacity of a whole hemithorax with extreme mediastinal retraction; the volume of the affected hemithorax is severely reduced with compensatory hyperinflation and mediastinal herniation of the contralateral lung (Fig. **9**) [6].

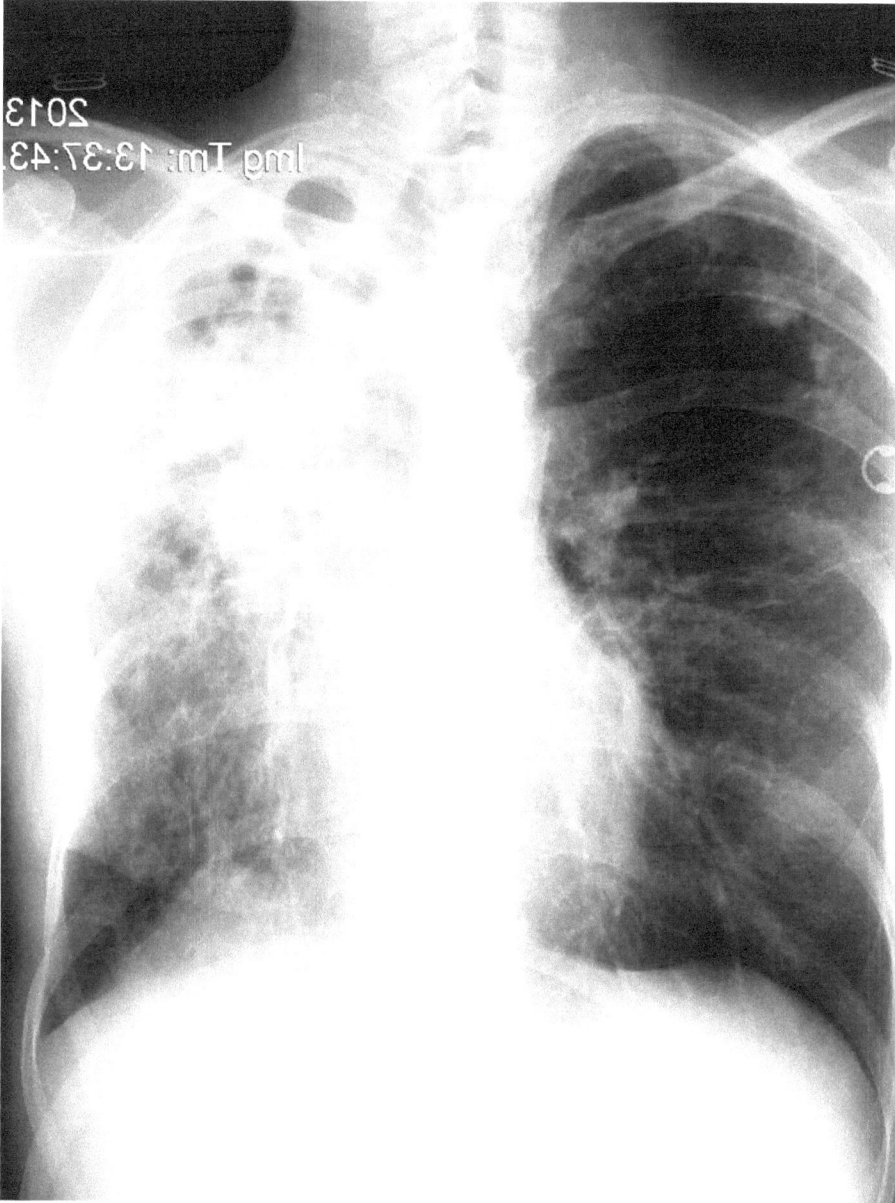

Fig. (9). Unilateral destroyed lung (cavitation in right upper lobe) with mediastinal and tracheal retraction and hyperinflation of the left lung.

Pulmonary mycetoma is secondary to a saprophytic fungal infection of a pre-existing lung cavity. TB is the cause of the pre-existing cavity in up to 80% of the cases of mycetoma, although in some cases, the cavity is secondary to other diseases. It consists of an intracavitary fungus ball that includes fungal hyphae, fibrin, mucus, and cellular debris. Most cases are secondary to *Aspergillus fumigatus*, but there can also be secondary to *Nocardia asteroides*, *Allescheria boydii*, and Mucorales. Radiographically, it presents as a ball-like lesion inside a cavity, partially surrounded by a radiolucent air crescent sign (Monod's sign, Fig. **10**) [7, 8].

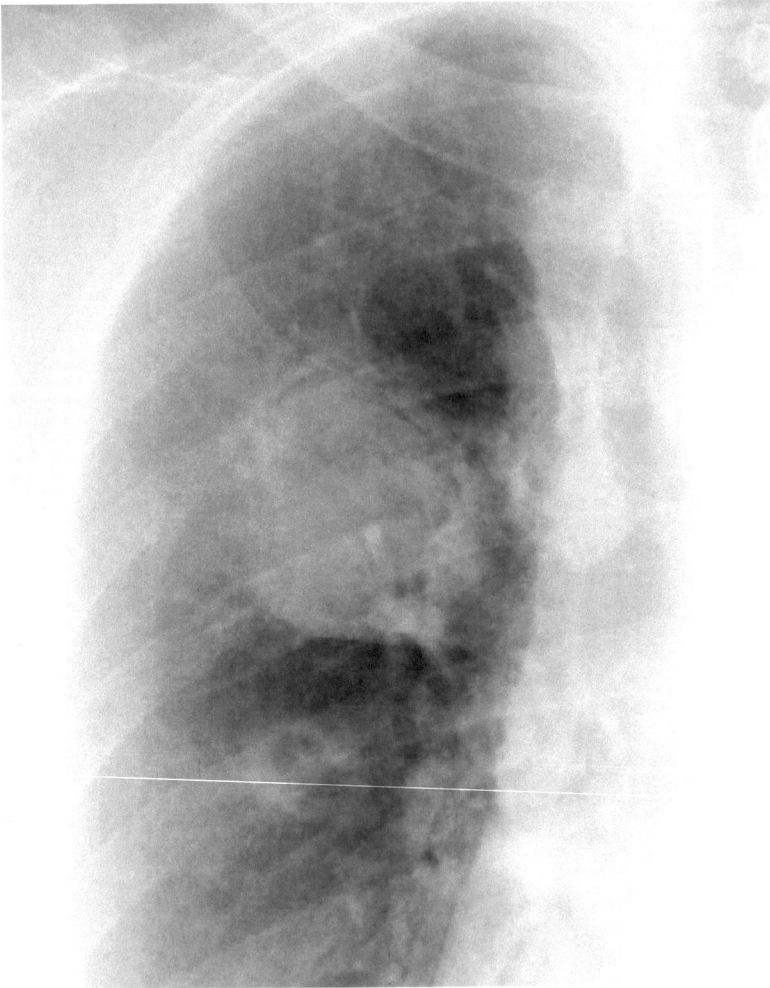

Fig. (10). Pulmonary mycetoma in a lung cavity (right upper lobe) with the air crescent sign (Monod´s sign).

IMAGING IN EXTRAPULMONARY TB

Although TB is mostly limited to the lungs, it can occur in any other tissue or organ, especially in the immunocompromised host.

TUBERCULOUS PERICARDITIS

Tuberculosis pericarditis is characterized by pericardial thickening and pericardial effusion. The chest x-rays show an enlarged cardiac silhouette (Figs. **11A** and **11B**); it frequently concurs with pleural effusion [9]. Echocardiography is the imaging modality of choice to assess the pericardium due to its non-invasiveness, its availability, and cost-effectiveness [10].

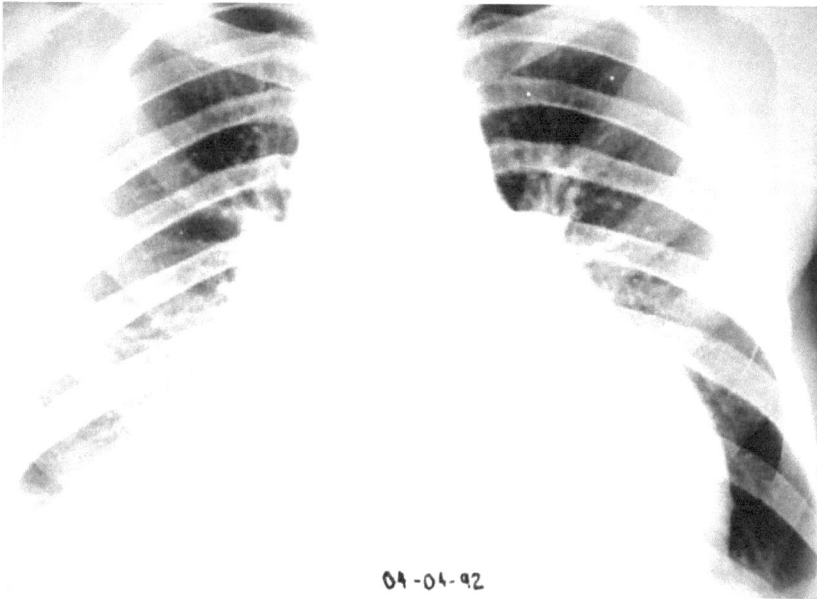

04-04-92

Fig. (11A). Pericardial tuberculous effusion concurrent with right-sided pleural effusion in a patient with co-infection with HIV.

CENTRAL NERVOUS SYSTEM TB

CNS involvement includes tuberculous meningitis, parenchymal tuberculomas, tuberculous abscesses, and miliary infiltrates.

The leptomeninges demonstrate intense, homogeneous enhancement, most prominent at the basal cisterns. The imaging modality of choice for meningeal TB is gadolinium-enhanced magnetic resonance imaging (MRI). A frequent complication of tuberculous meningitis is communicating hydrocephalus, secondary to blockage of the basal cisterns by inflammatory exudates [3].

The most frequent CNS parenchymal lesion is the tuberculoma; it may be solitary or multiple, most often found within the frontal and parietal lobes (Fig. **12**).

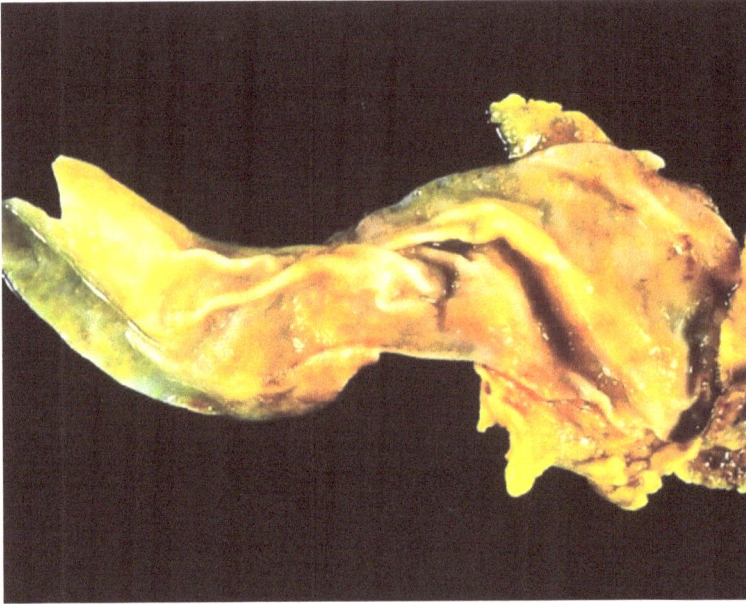

Fig. (11B). Thickened parietal pericardium from the patient in fig. (11A) removed during thoracoscopy; culture was reported positive for *M. tuberculosis*.

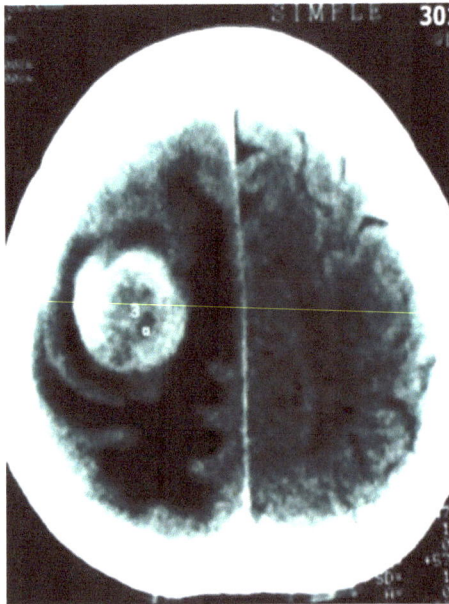

Fig. (12). Brain parenchymal tuberculoma with ring enhancement and marked edema.

Cerebral infarction is a frequent complication of TB meningitis; the basal ganglia is the most commonly affected site. Imaging in cerebral infarction reveals the thickness of the leptomeninges, where the exudate at the basal region encompasses the arteries leading to vascular obstruction and to inflammation that causes vasculitis and vasospasm [11].

SKELETAL TUBERCULOSIS

More than half of the cases of skeletal TB involve the spine, usually the lower thoracic and lumbar segments. If not treated, it progresses to vertebral collapse and anterior wedging, causing kyphosis and anterior extension of the abscess with a displacement of the anterior longitudinal ligament, also known as Pott´s disease (Figs. **13** and **14**).

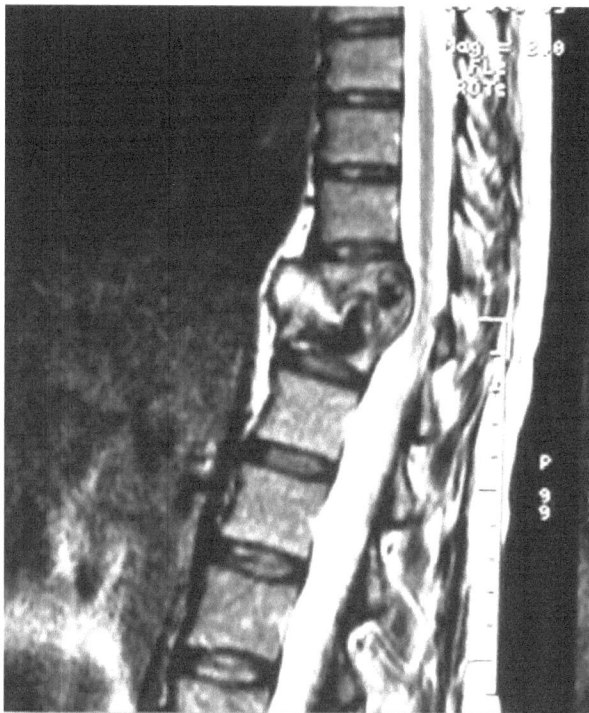

Fig. (13). MRI. Pott´s disease with vertebral collapse and anterior wedging and anterior extension of the abscess with a displacement of the anterior longitudinal ligament.

Tuberculosis arthritis is typically a monoarthritis that most frequently involves large weight-bearing joints, whose appearance is non-specific and indistinguishable from other infectious arthritides. Usually, there is osteoporosis, marginal erosions, and progressive narrowing of the joint space, a clinical presentation known as Phemister triad (Fig. **15**) [12].

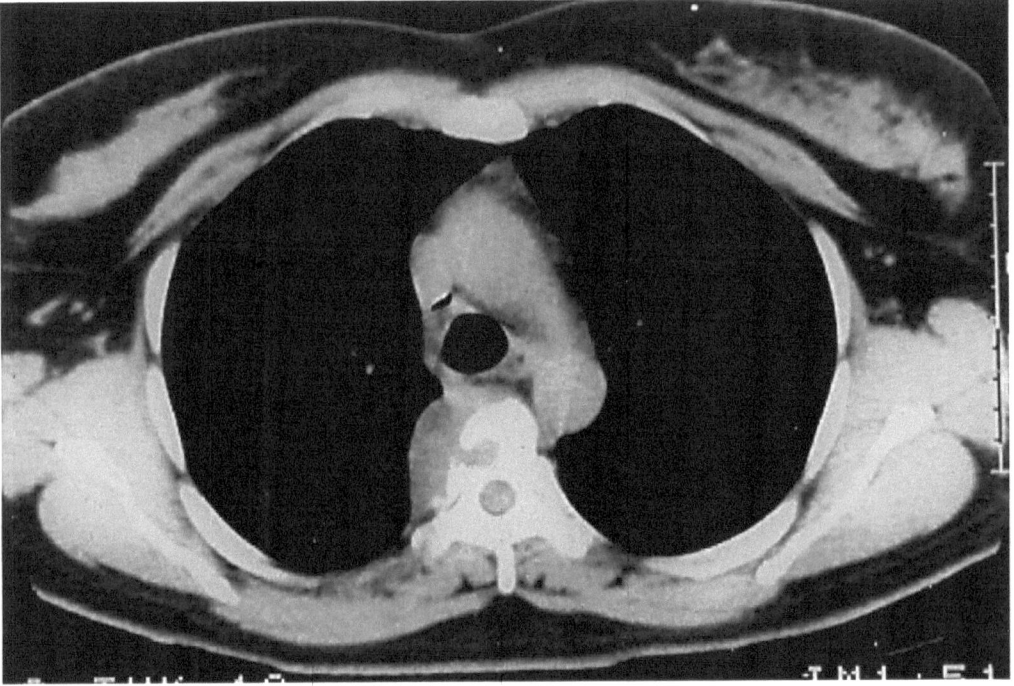

Fig. (14). Vertebral tuberculosis. Paravertebral abscess of a thoracic vertebra, with partial erosion of the vertebral body.

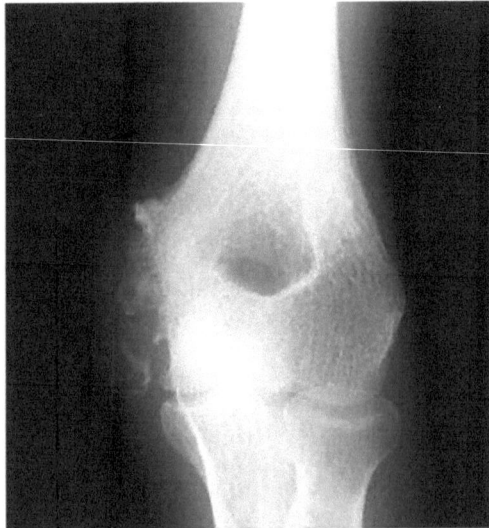

Fig. (15). Tuberculosis arthritis of the elbow with the destruction of the lateral epicondyle, edema of soft tissues, and narrowing of the joint space.

REFERENCES

[1]   Restrepo CS, Katre R, Mumbower A. Imaging manifestations of thoracic tuberculosis. Radiol Clin North Am 2016; 54(3): 453-73.
[http://dx.doi.org/10.1016/j.rcl.2015.12.007] [PMID: 27153783]

[2]   Curvo-Semedo L, Teixeira L, Caseiro-Alves F. Tuberculosis of the chest. Eur J Radiol 2005; 55(2): 158-72.
[http://dx.doi.org/10.1016/j.ejrad.2005.04.014] [PMID: 15905057]

[3]   Burrill J, Williams CJ, Bain G, Conder G, Hine AL, Misra RR. Tuberculosis: a radiologic review. Radiographics 2007; 27(5): 73-1255.
[http://dx.doi.org/10.1148/rg.275065176]

[4]   Sharma SK, Mukhopadhyay S, Arora R, Varma K, Pande JN, Khilnani GC. Computed tomography in miliary tuberculosis: comparison with plain films, bronchoalveolar lavage, pulmonary functions and gas exchange. Australas Radiol 1996; 40(2): 113-8.
[http://dx.doi.org/10.1111/j.1440-1673.1996.tb00363.x] [PMID: 8687341]

[5]   Miller WT, Miller WT Jr. Tuberculosis in the normal host: radiological findings. Semin Roentgenol 1993; 28(2): 109-18.
[http://dx.doi.org/10.1016/S0037-198X(05)80100-2] [PMID: 8516687]

[6]   Varona Porres D, Persiva O, Pallisa E, Andreu J. Radiological findings of unilateral tuberculous lung destruction. Insights Imaging 2017; 8(2): 271-7.
[http://dx.doi.org/10.1007/s13244-017-0547-4] [PMID: 28197882]

[7]   Golberg B. Radiological appearances in pulmonary aspergillosis. Clin Radiol 1962; 13: 106-14.
[http://dx.doi.org/10.1016/S0009-9260(62)80030-0] [PMID: 13899653]

[8]   Ramasamy A, Kadom Z, Dubrey SW. Pulmonary mycetoma. Br J Hosp Med (Lond) 2014; 75(11): 656.
[http://dx.doi.org/10.12968/hmed.2014.75.11.656] [PMID: 25383441]

[9]   Maclean KA, Becker AK, Chang SD, Harris AC. Extrapulmonary tuberculosis: imaging features beyond the chest. Can Assoc Radiol J 2013; 64(4): 319-24.
[http://dx.doi.org/10.1016/j.carj.2012.07.002] [PMID: 23267519]

[10]   Pérez-Casares A, Cesar S, Brunet-Garcia L. Echocardiographic evaluation of pericardial effusion and cardiac tamponade. Front Pediatr 2017; 64(4): 24-319.
[http://dx.doi.org/10.1016/j.carj.2012.07.002.]

[11]   Tai MS, Viswanathan S, Rahmat K, Nor HM, Kadir KAA, Goh KJ. Cerebral infarction pattern in tuberculous meningitis. Sci Rep 2016; 13: 6-38802.
[http://dx.doi.org/10.1038/srep38802]

[12]   Pattamapaspong N, Muttarak M, Sivasomboon C. Tuberculosis arthritis and tenosynovitis. Semin Musculoskelet Radiol 2011; 15(5): 459-69.
[http://dx.doi.org/10.1055/s-0031-1293492] [PMID: 22081281]

CHAPTER 6

Laboratory Diagnosis of Tuberculosis

Abstract: Although sputum microscopy remains the most widely used diagnostic method worldwide, given its low sensitivity (50-80%) and specificity (it does not distinguish *M. tuberculosis* from nontuberculous mycobacteria), more rapid, sensitive, and specific methods are required nowadays. Culture for mycobacteria continues to be the gold standard due to its higher sensitivity and specificity, and because it also allows the detection of strains resistant to antituberculosis drugs; however, even with liquid culture media, at least one month of processing is required to obtain results. Therefore, rapid genotyping methods (*e.g.*, Xpert and line-probe assays known as LPAs) have replaced phenotypic methods by allowing the identification of species and the presence of mutations associated with resistance in less than 24 hours. The Xpert, an automated real-time PCR system, can identify the presence of mutations associated with rifampin resistance in less than two hours, with a sensitivity higher than 70% in patients with negative microscopy. LPAs allow species identification and the presence of mutations associated with resistance to isoniazid, rifampin, fluoroquinolones, and second-line injectables in less than 24 hours. Progressively, the complete sequencing of the *Mycobacterium tuberculosis* genome has been integrated into the diagnostic protocol, allowing the identification of all mutations associated with resistance for all antituberculosis drugs. Phenotypic methods (microscopy and cultures) continue to play an essential role in the follow-up of patients who are already under treatment.

Keywords: Cultures, Diagnosis, Genome sequencing, LPA, MGIT, Microscopy, Tuberculosis, Xpert.

INTRODUCTION

Although the diagnosis of tuberculosis can be suspected clinically, it is essential to make a maximum efforts to achieve bacteriological confirmation, even more so at this time when drug resistance in new cases is widespread in countries with high TB burden. The definitive diagnosis of TB effort the isolation in a culture of *Mycobacterium tuberculosis* (MTB) or the identification of its DNA in mole-cular tests.

Rafael Laniado-Laborín

SMEAR MICROSCOPY

The ATS/CDC/IDSA guidelines recommend performing acid-fast bacillus (AFB) smear microscopy as an initial test in patients suspected of having pulmonary TB [1]. The sensitivity of an AFB smear microscopy 3 sample set is 54%, 65%, and 70% after the first, second, and third sample, respectively [2]. In some countries, to avoid loss of follow-up before diagnosis, it is recommended that patients produce two samples on the same day (instead of going to the health unit for 3 consecutive days) especially in rural areas with difficult access, since the third sample only contributes an extra 2-5% in the diagnosis [3]. The concentration of the sample (through centrifugation) increases the sensitivity of the method by 18% (using culture as a gold standard).

The quality of the sample is essential to increase the sensitivity of the test. Ideally, diagnostic samples should be obtained before starting treatment. It is recommended to obtain the samples after a night of fasting, in an area that reduces the risk of MTB transmission. Sputum samples should be collected in an expectoration induction booth with air extraction, or if this is not possible, in a space with proper ventilation that offers privacy. Plastic cups with screw caps that allow a hermetic seal is recommended (capacity 30-50 mL); the vials should be labeled (both the cup and the cap) with the patient identification data. An adequate sample must be at least 3-5 mL. To obtain another type of sample (abscess material, pleural fluid, cerebrospinal fluid, *etc.*), it is recommended to carry out an aseptic technique and transport the sample in a sterile container [4]. In patients who cannot expectorate spontaneously, sputum induction is recommended by nebulization of hypertonic saline solution over bronchoscopy, since sputum induction has a higher yield than endoscopy, has less risk and less cost. If bronchoscopy is needed, it is recommended to collect post-endoscopy samples for sputum smears and culture. Samples should be processed as soon as possible, especially if they are going to be cultured, to reduce the risk of contamination by oropharyngeal flora [1].

Conventional laboratory methods have a low sensitivity in the pediatric patient, given the paucibacillary nature of TB in children and the difficulty in obtaining adequate samples of sputum. In children, AFB smears are positive in only 10-15% of cases, and cultures in only 10-25% [5].

Traditionally gastric aspirate after a night of fasting has been considered the method of choice in infants to diagnose pulmonary TB tuberculosis. However, this implies having the patient hospitalized to carry out this invasive procedure, which hinders its realization in regions with a high burden of disease. Other less invasive methods, including the induction of sputum and nasopharyngeal aspiration, have already been evaluated, and the results suggest that both offer the same sensitivity as the gastric aspirate [6].

The most frequently used technique for microscopy is the Ziehl-Neelsen (ZN) method, also known as the acid-fast technique. The advantages of this method include that it is technically straightforward, requires just a few hours from the reception of the sample to the report, and it is very inexpensive. Its primary disadvantage is its low sensitivity (50-80%). The technique is based on the ability of the mycobacteria to fix the red dye (carbol-fuchsin) given the high lipid content of the bacterial wall (mycolic acid) and that it does not decolorate when the slide is irrigated with alcohol-acid (1% solution of hydrochloric acid in isopropyl alcohol). The slide is then stained again with methylene blue and examined under oil immersion. Mycobacteria appear colored red over a blue background. The Kinyoun method is similar to the ZN method, but the Kinyoun stain does not require heating of the carbol-fuchsin (Table 1) [7]. Fluorescent microscopy is, on average, 10% more sensitive than light microscopy. However, initially, it was not widely implemented since it required expensive (and potentially toxic) mercury vapor lamps and a dark room. The advent of LED (Light Emitting Diode) fluorescent microscopes that do not utilize mercury lamps or require a darkroom has increased its use; the fluorescent stain used for LED microscopy is Auramine O [8]. A study from India reported the sensitivity of LED microscopy, mercury vapor fluorescence, and light microscopy, respectively, as 83.1%, 82.4%, and 78.5%; reading time in this study was three times faster for LED microscopy than for light microscopy [9].

Table 1. Typical report of the microscopy results.

Results	Report
No AFB observed in 100 microscopic fields	Negative
1-9 AFB observed in 100 microscopic fields	Exact number of AFB seen
10-99 AFB observed in 100 microscopic fields	Positive 1+
1-10 AFB per field observed in 50 microscopic fields	Positive 2+
>10 AFB per field in 20 microscopic fields	Positive 3+

*Modified from Organización Panamericana de la Salud, 2008 [7].

MYCOBACTERIAL CULTURE (PHENOTYPIC METHOD)

It is still the gold standard for tuberculosis diagnosis (although eventually will be substituted by molecular techniques) and all patients should have at least one sample processed for culture. Unlike microscopy, that requires at least 5,000 bacilli/mL to obtain a positive test, cultures require only 10-100 bacilli/mL. There are two types of culture media used for the diagnosis of tuberculosis: solid and liquid media.

Solid media (there are different culture media, the Lowenstein-Jensen being the most frequently used) are inexpensive, have lower rate of contamination (<5%) but are less sensitive than liquid media and growth of mycobacteria can take up to 8-9 weeks. Liquid media have higher sensitivity (growth can be detected as soon as a couple of weeks) but are more expensive and have a higher rate of contamination (about 10%). The ATS/CDC/IDSA guidelines recommend culturing the sample in both types of media to benefit from each method (faster results with the liquid media and a safeguard against contamination with the solid media) [2]. There are automated systems for culture, such as the BACTEC MGIT 320 and 960 (Mycobacterial Growth Indicator Tube, Becton Dickinson). This system uses liquid media (Middlebrook 7 H9) with a fluorescent sensor to detect bacterial growth. Once growth is detected automatically by the equipment, species identification will take only 15 minutes using a lateral immunochromatography probe (*e.g.*, the SD TB Ag MPT 64 Rapid®, SD Bioline, Germany).

The gold standard for drug susceptibility testing (DST) for second-line drugs is still the agar proportion method. Its most significant disadvantage is its turnaround time (from 8-12 weeks). It will eventually be replaced by automated methods and molecular testing.

The MGIT system has been validated to perform drug susceptibility testing (DST) for first-line drugs (isoniazid, rifampin, ethambutol, pyrazinamide, and streptomycin) and second-line drugs using the proportion method as the gold standard, especially for fluoroquinolones, and second-line injectables. The agreement rates between the two methods for these drugs range from 90 to100%. With the indirect culture method (once there is growth in the liquid media, the strain is inoculated in media with antituberculosis drugs) turnaround time for DST results is 3-4 weeks. With the direct method (inoculating the sample directly in the media with antibiotics), the turnaround time is reduced to 10-14 days; however, the contamination rate with this method is unacceptably high (up to 15%).

One topic for controversy has been the reproducibility of the phenotypic DST; they are very reliable for isoniazid and rifampin and less reliable for streptomycin and ethambutol. The results of the tests for pyrazinamide are even more variable, especially with automated methods. DST for the second-line drugs should only be carried out by highly specialized laboratories. Of these, DST for fluoroquinolones (levofloxacin and moxifloxacin) and second-line injectables (kanamycin, amikacin, and capreomycin) are the most reliable [10 - 13].

MOLECULAR METHODS (GENOTYPIC METHODS)

Xpert MTB/RIF Assay

The GeneXpert diagnostic platform was launched in 2004. It is an automated, fully integrated system that performs the three processes required for a polymerase chain reaction (PCR): specimen preparation, amplification, and detection. It utilizes disposable cartridges (Xpert MTB/RIF) containing lyophilized reagents, buffers, and washing solutions. The system is the first point-of-care assay that can be used outside a mycobacteriology laboratory and it allows the identification of *Mycobacterium tuberculosis* complex as well as the mutations associated with rifampicin resistance through real-time PCR in less than two hours. There is no cross-reactivity with nontuberculous mycobacteria (NTM).

The system has excellent performance: overall sensitivity for MTB detection (using culture as the gold standard) is over 92%. For smear-negative and culture-positive patients, single test sensitivity is 72%; it increases to 90% if three samples are tested. The overall specificity is 99%. For rifampin, resistance sensitivity is 95%, and specificity is over 98%. Although HIV co-infection decreases the sensitivity of microscopy under 50%, it does not significantly affect the performance of the Xpert MTB/RIF system [14].

The World Health Organization (WHO) since 2013 has the following recommendations regarding the use of the Xpert MTB/RIF:

1. Xpert MTB/RIF may be used rather than conventional microscopy and culture as the initial diagnostic test in all adults suspected of having TB (conditional recommendation acknowledging resource implications, high-quality evidence).

2. Xpert MTB/RIF may be used rather than conventional microscopy and culture as the initial diagnostic test in all children suspected of having TB (conditional recommendation acknowledging resource implications, very low-quality evidence).

3. Xpert MTB/RIF should be used rather than conventional microscopy, culture, and DST as the initial diagnostic test in adults suspected of having MDR-TB or HIV-associated TB (strong recommendation, high-quality evidence).

4. Xpert MTB/RIF should be used rather than conventional microscopy, culture and DST as the initial diagnostic test in children suspected of having MDR-TB

or HIV associated TB (strong recommendation, very low-quality evidence) [15].

Aiming to improve the sensitivity of the Xpert MTB/RIF, the Xpert MTB/RIF Ultra (Xpert Ultra) assay was developed with the incorporation of two different multicopy amplification targets (IS6110 and IS1081) and improved cartridge design with a larger reaction chamber (50 μL PCR reaction in Ultra *vs*. 25 μL in the Xpert). The limit of detection (LOD) for the Ultra is 16 bacterial colony forming units (cfu/mL) *vs*. 114 cfu/mL for the Xpert. Ultra uses the same semi-quantitative categories used in the Xpert MTB/RIF assay (high, medium, low and very low) as well as a new category called "trace" that represents the lowest bacillary burden corresponds to the lowest bacillary burden for *M. tuberculosis* detection. If MTB is detected with a trace call, no interpretation can be made regarding rifampin resistance. The result is reported as MTB detected, trace, rifampin resistance indeterminate.

In a study that included 1,520 persons with signs and symptoms of TB, overall sensitivity of the Ultra was 5% higher than that of Xpert MTB/RIF but specificity, as expected with the higher sensitivity, was 3.2% lower. Sensitivity was especially higher (+17%) among smear-negative and culture-positive patients and in subject with HIV co-infection (+12%) [16].

In a recent multicenter study that included 1,753 patients, sensitivities for the Xpert Ultra and Xpert were 63% and 46% respectively in subjects with smear-negative and culture-positive sputum, and 90% and 77% for HIV+ culture-positive participants. Overall sensitivity was 88% for the Ultra *vs*. 83% for the Xpert in patients with a positive culture. Specificity was 96% for the Ultra *vs*. 98% for the Xpert. Both assays performed similarly in the detection of rifampin resistance [17].

Given the need for a rapid diagnostic test for multidrug-resistant tuberculosis (MDR-TB) and extensively resistant tuberculosis (XDR-TB), a new cartridge for the GeneXpert platform was developed to detect mutations associated with resistance to isoniazid, fluoroquinolones, and second-line injectables, directly from unprocessed sputum in less than two hours.

The new cartridge was tested in 308 patients with culture-proven tuberculosis, and the results were compared to phenotypic DST as a reference standard. Sensitivity for the assay was 83.3% for isoniazid, 88.4% for ofloxacin, 87.6% for moxifloxacin at a critical concentration of 0.5 μg/mL (and 96.2% at a critical concentration of 2.0 μg/mL), 71.4% for kanamycin and 70.7% for amikacin. The specificity of the assay was 94.3% or greater, except for moxifloxacin (84% at a critical concentration of 2.0 μg/mL). Compared to DNA sequencing as the reference standard, the sensitivities of the investigational assay for detecting mutations associated with resistance were 98.1% for isoniazid, 95.8% for fluoroquinolones, 92.7% for kanamycin, and 96.8% for amikacin; the specificity for all drugs was 99.6% or greater [18].

A Cochrane Review [19] assessed the accuracy of Xpert in extrapulmonary specimens. It included 66 unique studies that evaluated 16,213 samples for detection of extrapulmonary TB and rifampicin resistance. There was only one study that assessed the XpertMTB/RIF Ultra for TB meningitis. Pooled Xpert sensitivity (defined by culture) varied across different types of specimens (31% in pleural tissue to 97% in bone or joint fluid); Xpert sensitivity was > 80% in urine and bone or joint fluid and tissue. Pooled Xpert specificity (defined by culture) varied less than sensitivity (82% in bone or joint tissue to 99% in pleural fluid and urine). Xpert specificity was ≥ 98% in cerebrospinal fluid, pleural fluid, urine, and peritoneal fluid.

For cerebrospinal fluid the Xpert pooled sensitivity and specificity against culture were 71.1% (95%CI: 60.9% to 80.4%) and 98.0% (95%CI: 97.0% to 98.8%), respectively. For TB meningitis, the Ultra sensitivity and specificity against culture were 90% (95%CI: 55% to 100%) and 90% (95%CI: 83% to 95%), respectively.

For pleural fluid the Xpert pooled sensitivity and specificity against culture were 50.9% (95%CI: 39.7% to 62.8%) and 99.2% (95%CI: 98.2% to 99.7%), respectively.

For urine samples, the Xpert pooled sensitivity and specificity against culture were 82.7% (95%CI: 69.6% to 91.1%) and 98.7% (95%CI: 94.8% to 99.7%), respectively.

Regarding the Xpert testing for rifampicin resistance, its pooled sensitivity and specificity were 95.0% (95%CI: 89.7% to 97.9%) and 98.7% (95%CI: 97.8% to 99.4%), respectively [19].

Line-Probe Assays (LPAs)

Molecular technology based on nucleic acid amplification offers significant advantages over phenotypic diagnostic methods, including faster turnaround times, testing standardization, and the potential for high throughput. Line probe assays (LPAs) are tests that use PCR and reverse hybridization methods for the rapid detection of mutations associated with drug resistance. Line probe assays for tuberculosis are designed to identify *M. tuberculosis* complex and simultaneously detect mutations related to drug resistance.

LPAs For First-Line Drugs

Since 2008, the WHO approved the use of commercial LPAs for the identification of *M. tuberculosis* and the detection of mutations associated with drug-resistance. The WHO recommended at that time the INNO-LiPA Rif.TB assay (Innogenetics, Ghent, Belgium) and the GenoType MTBDRplus (version 1). Newer versions of LPAs have since been developed, including the Hain GenoType MTBDRplus version 2 and the Nipro NTM+MDRTB detection kit 2 (Tokyo, Japan).

The Hain version 1 and version 2 assays include rpoB probes to detect rifampicin resistance, kat G probes to detect mutations associated with high-level isoniazid resistance, and inhA probes to detect mutations usually associated with low-level isoniazid resistance. The Nipro LPA includes probes to identify also *M. avium, M. intracellulare* and *M. kansasii* [20].

The Hain test involves four steps:

1. decontamination of the specimen

2. isolation and amplification of DNA

3. detection of the amplification products by reverse hybridization

4. visualization using a streptavidin-conjugated alkaline phosphatase color reaction.

Each band on the test strip corresponds to a probe and determines the susceptibility of the specimen. A study evaluated the Nipro and the Hain version 2 LPAs and compared them with Hain version 1. There are no significant differences among the three assays for the detection of *M. tuberculosis* and mutations associated with resistance to rifampicin or isoniazid (using culture DST as reference standard). For rifampin resistance the sensitivity of the three assays, when testing directly from sputum, was over 96% with specificity over 97%; for indirect testing (from positive culture) the sensitivity was lower (91-92%) with specificity like that observed with the direct method.

The sensitivity for the detection of resistance to isoniazid directly from sputum was slightly lower (94-95%) with excellent specificity (about 97%). In indirect testing, sensitivity was lower (89%) with high specificity (98-99%).

A recent systematic review and meta-analysis [21] corroborated these results: sensitivity/specificity for rifampin resistance 96.7%/98.8%; for isoniazid resistance 90.2%/99.2%. For *M. tuberculosis* detection, sensitivity was 94% for smear-positive specimens and 44% for smear-negative samples [21].

The WHO published the following recommendations regarding the use of LPAs for first-line drugs [22]:

1. For patients with a sputum smear-positive specimen (direct testing) or a cultured isolate of *M. tuberculosis* (indirect testing) from either pulmonary or extrapulmonary sites, commercial molecular LPAs may be used as the initial test instead of phenotypic culture-based DST to detect resistance to rifampicin and isoniazid.

Testing directly from the sputum, LPAs detect 96% of patients whose MTB strain has mutations associated with rifampicin resistance and false-positive results for people whose TB is susceptible are rare (<2%). When testing directly from the sputum, LPAs dentifies 89% of patients with isoniazid resistance and false positives are also scarce (<2%). For MDR-TB, LPAs detect 93% of subjects with MDR-TB and false positives are rare (<1%).

1. LPAs are not recommended for the direct testing of smear-negative sputum specimens.

2. These recommendations do not eliminate the need for conventional culture-based DST, which is necessary to determine resistance to other anti-TB agents and to monitor the emergence of additional drug resistance.

3. Conventional culture-based DST for isoniazid may still be used to evaluate patients when the LPA result does not detect isoniazid resistance. Isoniazid resistance is highly correlated with rifampin resistance; therefore, a negative LPA test for isoniazid resistance in a patient with a positive LPA for rifampin resistance should be followed by phenotypic culture-based DST.

4. These recommendations apply to the use of LPA in children based on the generalization of data from adults.

LPAs for Second-Line Drugs

The Genotype® MTBDRsl LPA is a rapid diagnostic test (the assay can be completed in a single working day) for drug-resistant TB that detects mutations associated with drug resistance to second-line drugs (Table **2**). The MTBDRsl version 1.0 had probes to detect mutations related to fluoroquinolones (FQ), second-line injectables (SLI), and ethambutol resistance, and is no longer available. MTBDRsl version 2.0 detects the mutations in *M. tuberculosis* complex DNA associated with resistance to FQ (including ofloxacin, moxifloxacin, levofloxacin, and gatifloxacin) and SLI (including kanamycin, amikacin, and capreomycin) detected by version 1.0 as well as additional mutations. Version 1.0 identified mutations in the *gyrA* (associated with FQ resistance) and *rrs* (associated to SLI resistance). Version 2.0 includes additional probes for codons in the *gyrB* region and for codons in the *eis* promoter region (associated with SLI resistance), increasing the sensitivity of Version 2.0 (Fig. **1**). The presence of mutations in the gyrA region in Ver 2.0, associated with FQ resistance, has a high concordance with resistance to all drugs in that class. Likewise, mutations in the rrs region are related to resistance to both amikacin and kanamycin. Mutations in the gyrB and eis promoter do not necessarily imply resistance to all drugs within those classes. MDRTBsl can be performed directly on sputum, regardless if the sample is smear-positive or negative [23].

Table 2. Accuracy of MTBDRsl (version 2.0) for fluoroquinolone and second-line injectable drug resistance and XDR-TB, (direct testing on smear-positive specimens or smear negative sputum), phenotypic culture-based DST reference standard*.

Drug	Sensitivity (95%CI)	Specificity smear (95%CI)
Fluoroquinolones smear positive	97% (83-100%)	98% (93-100%)
Fluoroquinolones smear negative	80% (28-99%)	100% (40-100%)
Second-line injectables smear positive	89% (72-98%)	90% (84-95%)
Second-line injectables smear negative	80% (28-99%)	100% (40-100%)
XDR-TB smear positive	79% (49-95%)	97% (93-99%)
XDR-TB smear positive	50% (1-99%)	100% (59-100%)

*Modified from Theron G *et al.* [23].

In its 2016 guidelines, the WHO has the following recommendations for the second-line LPA (SL-LPA) in patients with confirmed rifampin-resistant or MDR-TB [24]:

GenoType **MTBDR*sl*** VER 2.0

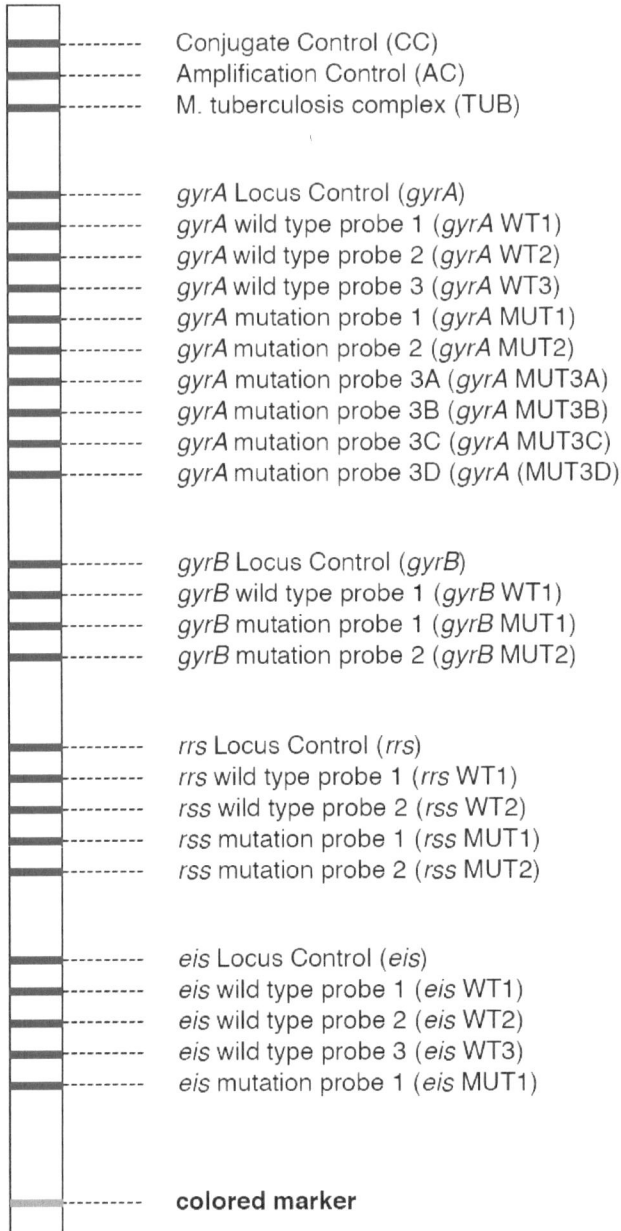

Conjugate Control (CC)
Amplification Control (AC)
M. tuberculosis complex (TUB)

gyrA Locus Control (*gyrA*)
gyrA wild type probe 1 (*gyrA* WT1)
gyrA wild type probe 2 (*gyrA* WT2)
gyrA wild type probe 3 (*gyrA* WT3)
gyrA mutation probe 1 (*gyrA* MUT1)
gyrA mutation probe 2 (*gyrA* MUT2)
gyrA mutation probe 3A (*gyrA* MUT3A)
gyrA mutation probe 3B (*gyrA* MUT3B)
gyrA mutation probe 3C (*gyrA* MUT3C)
gyrA mutation probe 3D (*gyrA* (MUT3D)

gyrB Locus Control (*gyrB*)
gyrB wild type probe 1 (*gyrB* WT1)
gyrB mutation probe 1 (*gyrB* MUT1)
gyrB mutation probe 2 (*gyrB* MUT2)

rrs Locus Control (*rrs*)
rrs wild type probe 1 (*rrs* WT1)
rss wild type probe 2 (*rss* WT2)
rss mutation probe 1 (*rss* MUT1)
rss mutation probe 2 (*rss* MUT2)

eis Locus Control (*eis*)
eis wild type probe 1 (*eis* WT1)
eis wild type probe 2 (*eis* WT2)
eis wild type probe 3 (*eis* WT3)
eis mutation probe 1 (*eis* MUT1)

colored marker

Fig. (1). Version 2.0 of the GenoType® MTBDRsl test (modified from Hain Life Sciences 2015).

1. SL-LPA may be used as the initial test, instead of phenotypic culture-based DST, to detect resistance to fluoroquinolones. This a conditional recommendation with moderate certainty of the evidence for the direct test on sputum samples and low certainty for the indirect test from *M. tuberculosis* cultures. Indeterminate results for the SL-LPAs are more frequent when testing smear-negative sputum specimens.

2. SL-LPA may be used as the initial test, instead of phenotypic culture-based DST, to detect resistance to the second-line injectable drugs. This is also a conditional recommendation with low certainty for direct testing on sputum samples and very low certainty for indirect testing from cultures. These recommendations apply to the use of SL-LPA for testing sputum specimens and culture specimens from both pulmonary and extrapulmonary sites. Direct testing of sputum allows for earlier diagnosis.

3. SL-LPA can be used for diagnosis of XDR-TB; however, the accuracy for detecting resistance to fluoroquinolones and SLIs differs, and therefore, the accuracy of a diagnosis of XDR-TB overall is reduced.

4. Conventional phenotypic DST capacity is necessary to confirm resistance to other drugs and to monitor the emergence of additional drug resistance.

5. Mutations detected by SL-LPA are highly correlated with phenotypic resistance to ofloxacin and levofloxacin. The correlation with phenotypic resistance to moxifloxacin and gatifloxacin is unclear, and phenotypic DST results, best guide the inclusion of moxifloxacin or gatifloxacin in a regimen.

6. Mutations detected by SL-LPA are highly correlated with phenotypic resistance to SLI.

7. These recommendations apply to children with confirmed rifampicin-resistant TB or MDR-TB based on the generalization of data from adults.

OTHER DIAGNOSTIC METHODS

Lateral-Flow LAM Test

Mycobacterial lipoarabinomannan (LAM) is an antigen present in the mycobacterial cell wall that is released by metabolically active or degenerating mycobacteria that can be detected in the urine of people with active TB disease and has the advantage of being easier to collect than sputum without the risk of infection associated with sputum collection.

The lateral flow urine lipoarabinomannan test (LF-LAM) is a commercial assay for the diagnosis of active TB (Alere DetermineTM TB LAM Ag®, Alere Inc, Waltham, MA, USA). The test is performed by applying 60 μL of urine to the test strip and incubating it for 25 minutes. The test is inspected by eye to determine if there are any visible band and grading its intensity by comparing it with that of the bands on a reference card. The card has four lines going from low (line 1) to high (line 4) intensity lines.

Conversely to other traditional TB tests in patients with HIV, meta-analysis have shown a higher sensitivity of the LF-LAM in subjects with HIV-TB co-infection, which increases with lower CD4 counts. This higher sensitivity could be explained by a higher antigen load and a greater frequency of disseminated disease in HIV patients, allowing increased antigen levels in urine. Compared with a microbiological reference standard in HIV-infected patients with microbiologically proven TB, the pooled sensitivity of the LF-LAM assay was 44% (95% CI 31-60%), and the pooled specificity was 92% (95% CI 83-96%). In HIV-positive individuals with tuberculosis, sensitivity for those with <100 CD4 cells was 56% (95%Cr 41-70%) with 90% specificity (95%Cr 81-95%).

In 2015 the WHO issued the following recommendations for the LF-LAM assay [25]:

1. Except for persons with HIV infection with low CD4 counts or who are seriously ill (respiratory rate > 30/min, temperature > 39°C, heart rate > 120/min and unable to walk unaided.) LF-LAM should not be used for the diagnosis of TB. This is a strong recommendation, despite the low quality of evidence.

2. LF-LAM may be used to assist in the diagnosis of TB in HIV positive adult in-patients with signs and symptoms of TB (pulmonary and/or extrapulmonary) who have a CD4 cell count less than or equal to 100 cells/μL, or HIV positive patients who are seriously ill, regardless of CD4 count or with unknown CD4 count. This is a conditional recommendation due to the low quality of evidence. This recommendation also applies to HIV positive children with signs and symptoms of TB (pulmonary or extrapulmonary) based on the generalization of data from adults.

3. LF-LAM should not be used as a screening test for TB. Due to its low sensitivity, the LF-LAM is deemed unsuitable as a general screening test. This is a strong recommendation despite the low quality of evidence.

TB-LAMP Method

Loop-mediated isothermal amplification is a straightforward technique for amplifying DNA that requires minimal laboratory infrastructure and can be used at the point of care. There is a commercial manual assay (Loopamp™ *Mycobacterium tuberculosis* complex [MTBC], Eiken Chemical Company Tokyo, Japan) to detect *M. tuberculosis* directly from sputum based on the TB-LAMP technique that takes less than an hour to perform and can be directly visually read under ultraviolet light. The reaction generates large amounts of amplicons that can be detected using DNA fluorescent binding dyes (*e.g.*, SYBR green).

In 2016 the WHO published the following recommendations regarding the use of the TB-LAMP technique:

1. TB-LAMP may be used as a replacement test for sputum-smear microscopy to diagnose pulmonary TB in adults with signs and symptoms consistent with TB. This is a conditional recommendation due to the very low quality of the evidence.

2. TB-LAMP may be used as a follow-on test to smear microscopy in adults with signs and symptoms consistent with pulmonary TB, especially when further testing of sputum smear-negative specimens is necessary (conditional recommendation, very low-quality evidence).

The WHO guideline emphasizes that this technique should not replace the use of rapid molecular tests for identification of M tuberculosis and resistance to rifampin. These recommendations are extrapolated to the use of the TB-LAMP technique in children, based on the generalization of data from adults.

A systematic review showed that sensitivity for the TB-LAMP ranged from 77.7% to 80.3%. When sensitivity differences were pooled across studies, TB-LAMP ranged from being 7.1% to 13.2% more sensitive than sputum-smear microscopy. Specificity in individual studies ranged from 90% to 99%. When specificity differences were pooled across studies, TB-LAMP performed similarly to sputum-smear microscopy; pooled specificity differences ranged from -1.8% to -1.3% [26].

TrueNat MTB

The TrueNat MTB and MTB Plus assays and the rifampicin-resistance detection reflex assay (Truenat MTB-RIF Dx) (Molbio Diagnostics, India) is a two-step real-time micro-PCR for detection of *M. tuberculosis* and rifampicin resistance a patient's sputum specimen. The assays use battery-operated devices to extract, amplify and confirm the presence TB infections with minimal user input. As with the Xpert MTB/RIF the test can be carried out by a technician with minimal training. The assay reports the results in less than one hour. If the test detects *M. tuberculosis*, another aliquot of extracted DNA may be used to run the MTB-Rif Dx assay to detect the presence of rifampin resistance [24].

In a recent study the overall performance of the test with MGIT culture as gold standard, sensitivity of RT PCR/TrueNAT and Genexpert was 94.7% (CI:89.8–97.6%) and 96.0% (CI: 91.5–98.5%), respectively. Amongst the smear positive cases RT-PCR/TrueNAT and GeneXpert showed a sensitivity of 99% (CI:94.9%–99.8%) and 100% (98.6%–100.0%), respectively [27].

Regarding the Truenat assay the WHO has the two following recommendations [24]:

1. In adults and children with signs and symptoms of pulmonary TB, the Truenat MTB or MTB Plus may be used as an initial diagnostic test for TB (conditional recommendation, low certainty of evidencefor test accuracy).

2. In adults and children with signs and symptoms of pulmonary TB and a Truenat MTB or MTB Plus positive result, Truenat MTB-RIF Dx may be used as an initial test for rifampicin resistance (conditional recommendation, very low certainty of evidence for test accuracy).

WHOLE GENOME SEQUENCING FOR THE DIAGNOSIS OF TUBERCULOSIS

Whole Genome Sequencing (WGS) is the process of reading the complete DNA sequence of an organism's genetic material. The genome of *M. tuberculosis* (MTB) is a sequence of four million nucleotides. Although the Xpert and the LPA genotypic assays are fast and are readily available in both high-income and low-income countries, these assays only screen a small number of genetic loci commonly associated with drug resistance. WGS allows the screening of known resistance-associated loci while also providing opportunities to characterize other loci as predictive of resistance or not. The characterization of all existing mutations offers advantages over the Xpert and the LPA's assays. Drug-susceptibility testing (DST) based on WGS can be done for drugs not included in the traditional phenotypic drug susceptibility tests or the commercial molecular assay, including novel drugs like bedaquiline and delamanid [28].

WGS of MTB allows not only the simultaneous identification of all known resistance mutations but also of markers with which transmission can be monitored, and provides resolution superior to that of other current methods, such as spoligotyping and mycobacterial interspersed repetitive-unit–variable-number tandem repeat (MIRU-VNTR) analysis for strain genotyping.

Traditionally WGS has been carried from positive cultures of MTB, which requires waiting for at least a couple of weeks for bacterial growth. Although there have also been attempts to perform WGS directly from sputum, results have been variable. There are reports that it is possible to run accurate sequencing of *M. tuberculosis* genomes directly from clinical samples. Identification of known resistance mutations within a week offers the prospect for personalized rather than standardized empirical treatment of DR-TB, leading to improved outcomes [29].

Full WGS diagnostics could be generated in 6 to 10 days, three weeks faster than conventional DST at a lower cost than that of existing diagnostic workflows [30].

WGS can provide the near-complete genome of MTB in a sample, while targeted Next-generation sequencing (NGS) can generate MTB sequence data at specific genetic loci of interest. Since drug resistance in MTB is mainly conferred through point mutations in specific gene targets, targeted NGS offers great promise for the rapid diagnosis of DR-TB [31].

REFERENCES

[1]   Jamil SM, Oren E, Garrison GW, *et al.* Diagnosis of tuberculosis in adults and children. Ann Am Thorac Soc 2017; 14(2): 275-8.
       [PMID: 28146376]

[2]   Lewinsohn DM, Leonard MK, LoBue PA, *et al.* Official american thoracic society/infectious diseases society of america/centers for disease control and prevention clinical practice guidelines: diagnosis of tuberculosis in adults and children. Clin Infect Dis 2017; 64(2): e1-e33.
       [http://dx.doi.org/10.1093/cid/ciw694] [PMID: 27932390]

[3]   Mase SR, Ramsay A, Ng V, *et al.* Yield of serial sputum specimen examinations in the diagnosis of pulmonary tuberculosis: a systematic review. Int J Tuberc Lung Dis 2007; 11(5): 485-95.
       [PMID: 17439669]

[4]   Farga V, Caminero JA. Tuberculosis editorial mediterráneo. 3ra . Santiago de Chile 2011; pp. 109-38.
       ISBN: 978-956-220-312-8.

[5]   Thomas TA, Heysell SK, Moodley P, *et al.* Intensified specimen collection to improve tuberculosis diagnosis in children from Rural South Africa, an observational study. BMC Infect Dis 2014; 14: 11.
       [http://dx.doi.org/10.1186/1471-2334-14-11] [PMID: 24400822]

[6]   Laniado-Laborín R. Alternativas actuales para la confirmación diagnóstica de tuberculosis en pacientes pediátricos. Neumol Pediatr 2015; 10(4): 174-8.

[7]   Organización Panamericana de la Salud. Manual para el diagnóstico Normas y Guía Técnica Bacteriológico de la tuberculosis. OPS 2008.

[8]   Singhal R, Myneedu VP. Microscopy as a diagnostic tool in pulmonary tuberculosis. Int J Mycobacteriol 2015; 4(1): 1-6.

[http://dx.doi.org/10.1016/j.ijmyco.2014.12.006] [PMID: 26655191]

[9] Bhalla M, Sidiq Z, Sharma PP, Singhal R, Myneedu VP, Sarin R. Performance of light-emitting diode fluorescence microscope for diagnosis of tuberculosis. Int J Mycobacteriol 2013; 2(3): 174-8.
[http://dx.doi.org/10.1016/j.ijmyco.2013.05.001] [PMID: 26785987]

[10] Krüüner A, Yates MD, Drobniewski FA. Evaluation of MGIT 960-based antimicrobial testing and determination of critical concentrations of first- and second-line antimicrobial drugs with drug-resistant clinical strains of *Mycobacterium tuberculosis*. J Clin Microbiol 2006; 44(3): 811-8.
[http://dx.doi.org/10.1128/JCM.44.3.811-818.2006] [PMID: 16517859]

[11] Lin SYG, Desmond E, Bonato D, Gross W, Siddiqi S. Multicenter evaluation of bactec mgit 960 system for second-line drug susceptibility testing of *Mycobacterium tuberculosis* complex. J Clin Microbiol 2009; 47(11): 3630-4.
[http://dx.doi.org/10.1128/JCM.00803-09] [PMID: 19741086]

[12] Said HM, Kock MM, Ismail NA, *et al.* Comparison between the BACTEC MGIT 960 system and the agar proportion method for susceptibility testing of multidrug resistant tuberculosis strains in a high burden setting of South Africa. BMC Infect Dis 2012; 12: 369.
[http://dx.doi.org/10.1186/1471-2334-12-369] [PMID: 23259765]

[13] Kim H, Seo M, Park YK, *et al.* Evaluation of mgit 960 system for the second-line drugs susceptibility testing of *Mycobacterium tuberculosis*. Tuberc Res Treat 2013; 2013: 108401.
[http://dx.doi.org/10.1155/2013/108401] [PMID: 23606961]

[14] World Health Organization. Xpert MTB/RIF implementation manual: technical and operational 'how-to'; practical considerations. WHO/HTM/TB/2014.1. ISBN: 978 92 4 150670 0. 2014.

[15] World Health Organization 2013. Automated real-time nucleic acid amplification technology for rapid and simultaneous detection of tuberculosis and rifampicin resistance: Xpert MTB/RIF assay for the diagnosis of pulmonary and extrapulmonary TB in adults and children. Policy update. WHO/HTM/TB/2013.16. ISBN: 978 92 4 150633 5.

[16] World Health Organization 2017. WHO meeting report of a technical expert consultation: non-inferiority analysis of Xpert MTF/RIF Ultra compared to Xpert MTB/RIF. Geneva: World Health Organization; 2017 (WHO/HTM/TB/2017.04). Licence: CC BY-NCSA 3.0 IGO.

[17] Dorman SE, Schumacher SG, Alland D, *et al.* study team. Xpert MTB/RIF Ultra for detection of *Mycobacterium tuberculosis* and rifampicin resistance: a prospective multicentre diagnostic accuracy study. Lancet Infect Dis 2018; 18(1): 76-84.
[http://dx.doi.org/10.1016/S1473-3099(17)30691-6] [PMID: 29198911]

[18] Xie YL, Chakravorty S, Armstrong DT, *et al.* Evaluation of a Rapid Molecular Drug-Susceptibility Test for Tuberculosis. N Engl J Med 2017; 377(11): 1043-54.
[http://dx.doi.org/10.1056/NEJMoa1614915] [PMID: 28902596]

[19] Kohli M, Schiller I, Dendukuri N, *et al.* Xpert® MTB/RIF assay for extrapulmonary tuberculosis and rifampicin resistance. Cochrane Database Syst Rev 2018; 8(8): CD012768.
[http://dx.doi.org/10.1002/14651858.CD012768.pub2] [PMID: 30148542]

[20] World Health Organization 2016-1. The use of molecular line probe assay for the detection of resistance to isoniazid and rifampicin: policy update. WHO/HTM/TB/2016.12. ISBN 978 92 4 151126 1.

[21] Nathavitharana RR, Cudahy PGT, Schumacher SG, Steingart KR, Pai M, Denkinger CM. Accuracy of line probe assays for the diagnosis of pulmonary and multidrug-resistant tuberculosis: a systematic review and meta-analysis. Eur Respir J 2017; 49.
[http://dx.doi.org/10.1183/13993003.01075-2016] [PMID: 1601075]

[22] World Health Organization 2016. The use of molecular line probe assay for the detection of resistance to isoniazid and rifampicin: policy update. ISBN 978 92 4 151126 1.

[23] Theron G, Peter J, Richardson M, Warren R, Dheda K, Steingart KR. GenoType® MTBDRsl assay for

resistance to second-line anti-tuberculosis drugs. Cochrane Database Syst Rev 2016; 9(9): CD010705.
[http://dx.doi.org/10.1002/14651858.CD010705.pub3] [PMID: 27605387]

[24]   WHO consolidated guidelines on tuberculosis. Module 3: diagnosis – rapid diagnostics for tuberculosis detection. Geneva: World Health Organization; 2020. Licence: CC BY-NC-SA 3.0 IGO.

[25]   World Health Organization 2015. The use of lateral flow urine lipoarabinomannan assay (LF-LAM) for the diagnosis and screening of active tuberculosis in people living with HIV. Policy guidance. WHO/HTM/TB/2015.25ISBN 978 92 4 150963.

[26]   World Health Organization 2016-3. The use of loop-mediated isothermal amplification (TB-LAMP) for the diagnosis of pulmonary tuberculosis. Policy guidance. WHO/HTM/TB/2016.11. ISBN 978 92 4 151118 6.

[27]   Nikam C, Kazi M, Nair C, *et al.* Evaluation of the Indian TrueNAT micro RT-PCR device with GeneXpert for case detection of pulmonary tuberculosis. Int J Mycobacteriol 2014; 3(3): 205-10.
[http://dx.doi.org/10.1016/j.ijmyco.2014.04.003] [PMID: 26786489]

[28]   Walker TM, Kohl TA, Omar SV, *et al.* Modernizing Medical Microbiology (MMM) Informatics Group. Whole-genome sequencing for prediction of *Mycobacterium tuberculosis* drug susceptibility and resistance: a retrospective cohort study. Lancet Infect Dis 2015; 15(10): 1193-202.
[http://dx.doi.org/10.1016/S1473-3099(15)00062-6] [PMID: 26116186]

[29]   Brown AC, Bryant JM, Einer-Jensen K, *et al.* Rapid whole-genome sequencing of *Mycobacterium tuberculosis* isolates directly from clinical samples. J Clin Microbiol 2015; 53(7): 2230-7.
[http://dx.doi.org/10.1128/JCM.00486-15] [PMID: 25972414]

[30]   Pankhurst LJ, Del Ojo Elias C, Votintseva AA, *et al.* Rapid, comprehensive, and affordable mycobacterial diagnosis with whole-genome sequencing: a prospective study. Lancet Respir Med 2016; 4(1): 49-58.
[http://dx.doi.org/10.1016/S2213-2600(15)00466-X] [PMID: 26669893]

[31]   World Health Organization. The use of next-generation sequencing technologies for the detection of mutations associated with drug resistance in *Mycobacterium tuberculosis* complex: technical guide. 2018.

CHAPTER 7

Tuberculosis in Special Situations: Liver and Renal Disease, Pregnancy, Extrapulmonary Tuberculosis, Tuberculosis in Immunosuppressed Individuals other than HIV, Tuberculosis, and Diabetes

Abstract: Although the underlying general principles of management of tuberculosis are the same for all cases, there are certain special situations in which the treatment regimen must be modified.

Uremia and post-renal transplant are both risk factors for tuberculosis due to the underlying immunodeficiency. Patients undergoing dialysis have a 10-25-fold higher risk of developing the disease than the general population.

Many antituberculosis drugs are hepatotoxic. If aspartate aminotransferase (AST) and alanine aminotransferase (ALT) are increased more than three times the upper limit of normal in the presence of symptoms of hepatitis or >5 times the upper limit of normal, even if the patient is asymptomatic, all hepatotoxic drugs should be discontinued.

First-line drugs (HREZ) are safe during pregnancy, and regimen doses and duration are the same as in non-pregnant individuals. Pyridoxine (50 mg, vitamin B6) should be added to the regimen to prevent neuropathy in the mother and seizures in the fetus.

There is an increased risk of progression to active TB in subjects with latent infection TB and diabetes in comparison with the infected nondiabetic population. Also, outcomes for patients with TB and diabetes are worse than for TB patients without diabetes, and diabetes also increases the risk of drug-resistant TB.

Risk factors for extrapulmonary TB (EPTB) include advanced age, female gender, immunosuppression (including HIV) and chronic comorbidities. Symptoms and signs are usually non-specific, and except for miliary forms, the chest radiograph might be normal; therefore, the diagnosis of EPTB is frequently delayed with the consequent increase in morbidity and mortality.

Keywords: Diabetes, Hepatotoxicity, HIV, Pregnancy, Renal failure, Tuberculosis.

Rafael Laniado-Laborín

INTRODUCTION

Although the underlying general principles of management of tuberculosis are the same, regardless of the clinical context, there are certain special situations in which the treatment regimen must be modified [1, 2]. This chapter includes the most common comorbidities and unique circumstances that require an individual approach for diagnosis and treatment.

CHRONIC RENAL FAILURE

Uremia and post-renal transplant are both risk factors for tuberculosis due to the underlying immunodeficiency. Patients undergoing dialysis have a 10-25-fold higher risk of developing the disease than the general population.

The general strategy for antituberculosis drugs that are cleared by the kidney is to increase the interval between dosing, rather than to decrease the dose. Of the first-line drugs, rifampin (R), isoniazid (H), and pyrazinamide (Z) are metabolized in the liver and excreted mainly by the biliary route and can be administered safely in chronic renal failure. R and H can be administered daily while Z and ethambutol (EMB) are recommended at regular doses but only three times a week. Of the second-line drugs, moxifloxacin (Mfx), ethionamide (ETA), para-aminosalicylic acid (PAS), linezolid (LZD) and clofazimine (CFZ) can be administered daily at usual doses. In contrast, cycloserine (CS), levofloxacin (LFX), and the second line injectables must be administered at regular doses but only three times per week. Since streptomycin (S) and the second line injectables (amikacin [Am], kanamycin [Km] and capreomycin [Cp]) are excreted exclusively by the kidneys, its use should be avoided if possible since there may be some accumulation of the second line injectables increasing the risk of ototoxicity and vestibular dysfunction. Serum drug concentrations, when available, can be used to verify that adequate drug concentrations are achieved. Medications should be administered immediately following hemodialysis [1, 2].

CHRONIC LIVER DISEASE

Many antituberculosis drugs are hepatotoxic. Of the first-line drugs, H is the most frequent cause of antituberculosis drug-induced hepatitis. In patients with previously normal liver function, hepatitis is usually reversible if the medicines are stopped immediately after the appearance of signs and symptoms (tiredness, jaundice, the elevation of liver enzymes). R is associated more with cholestatic jaundice than to hepatitis but can potentiate H induced-hepatitis. Although Z induced hepatitis is less frequent than that associated to H, is usually more severe and can worsen even after stopping the drug; Z, it is considered the most hepatotoxic antituberculosis drug and should never be used again in a patient of hepatitis. Of the second-line drugs, ETA, MFX, and PAS are also hepatotoxic.

Although carriers of hepatitis B and C infection and alcoholics potentially represent a higher risk of hepatotoxicity, they can be treated by avoiding hepatotoxic drugs (Z among the first-line drugs); since these patients do not receive Z, treatment with HRE should be prolonged to 9 months. Monthly monitoring of liver function must be carried out in this population. It is important to remember that up to 15% of patients receiving the first-line regimen (HRZE) develop minor transient elevation of liver enzymes (alanine aminotransferase [ALT] and aspartate aminotransferase [AST]) and it is not necessary to suspend the treatment.

If AST and ALT are elevated but <3 times the upper limit of normal (± 40 IU) and there no jaundice (total bilirubin <3 mg/dL), it is not necessary to stop treatment, but weekly monitoring of liver function must be carried out. If AST and ALT are elevated more than 3 times the upper limit of normal in the presence of symptoms of hepatitis, or >5 times the upper limit of normal even if the patient is asymptomatic, all hepatotoxic drugs should be stopped.

In patients with very severe chronic disease, further liver damage could be life-threatening, and all hepatotoxic drugs should be avoided, and a regimen can be completed with some of the following drugs: LFX, EMB, a second-line injectable, CS, LZD, bedaquiline (BDQ) and CFZ.

If treatment was stopped because there were not enough non-hepatotoxic drugs to build an efficient regimen, a regimen without hepatotoxic drugs could be restarted once the liver enzymes normalize, adding one potentially hepatotoxic drug at a time. If this regimen is tolerated, other potentially hepatotoxic drugs (if needed) can be reintroduced, one at a time. These patients should be closely monitored with liver function tests (weekly) for at least a month after the reintroduction of the potentially hepatotoxic drugs. If the reinstatement of a drug produces a relapse of hepatitis, the drug must be permanently eliminated from the regimen [3].

PREGNANCY

Tuberculosis is not associated with a statistically significant increase in congenital malformations, although there is evidence of prematurity, fetal growth retardation with low birth weight and increased perinatal mortality [4]. During the pregnant patient clinical evaluation, X-rays should preferably be deferred until the end of the first trimester.

First-line drugs (HREZ) are safe during pregnancy, and regimen doses and duration are the same as in non-pregnant women. Pyridoxine (50 mg, vitamin B6) should be added to the regimen to prevent neuropathy in the mother and seizures in the fetus.

Rifampin is a potent inducer of hepatic enzymes and decreases the effectiveness of oral contraceptives, and an alternative method of contraception should be recommended. Treatment of drug-resistant TB during pregnancy can be challenging. Several drugs used for treating MDR-TB are teratogenic, or their safety during pregnancy is unknown. Females of childbearing age with MDR-TB should be advised to avoid pregnancy through effective forms of contraception, like intrauterine devices or implantable hormonal contraceptives.

Aminoglycosides are the only TB drugs that have well-documented teratogenicity and are contraindicated during pregnancy since they are ototoxic and produce fetal deafness. Ethionamide/prothionamide and fluoroquinolones are contrain-dicated during pregnancy. Ethionamide has been reported as teratogenic, and fluoroquinolones have been reported to cause an injury to the cartilage growth in dogs. However, both have been used accidentally during pregnancy without reports of teratogenicity [5, 6]. If possible, those drugs should be avoided during pregnancy, at least during the first trimester.

Most antituberculosis drugs appear in breast milk at low levels. If the mother is receiving H, CS, and ETA, 50 mg of pyridoxine (vitamin B6) should be added to the regimen, and the infant should also receive pyridoxine (6.5 mg/day). The concentration of antituberculosis drugs in breast milk is too low to be considered adequate for treatment or prevention of tuberculosis in the infant.

There are two situations regarding the newborn and maternal TB: a) it is necessary to rule out congenital TB and b) what measures should be implemented to prevent infection of the infant.

a. Congenital TB is extremely rare and occurs when the mother has disseminated tuberculosis (or TB of the reproductive system) and has not received treatment. The infant presents with fever, irritability, visceromegaly, lymphadenopathy, tachypnea, and abnormal chest x-rays. If congenital TB is suspected, gastric aspirate collection and lumbar puncture should be carried out to obtain samples for laboratory testing. If congenital TB is confirmed, treatment should be started immediately based on the mother culture isolate susceptibility.

b. Prevention of infection in the newborn. If the mother is still infectious (or it is not possible to rule it out), the infant should be separated from the mother until she is not contagious. Preventive treatment is recommended if the newborn is healthy and has a normal chest radiograph. The drug of choice depends on the mother's culture drug susceptibility tests. The infant should be monitored closely (weekly) to rule out active disease [1, 2].

TUBERCULOSIS, AND DIABETES

Since diabetes is associated with a higher risk of active tuberculosis, the increased global burden of diabetes might counter the worldwide efforts to control the TB epidemic [7, 8].

There is an increased risk of progression to active TB in subjects with latent infection TB and diabetes in comparison with the infected non-diabetic population. Also, outcomes for patients with TB and diabetes are worse than for TB patients without diabetes [9], and diabetes also increases the risk of drug-resistant TB.

Patients with diabetes and tuberculosis have delayed culture conversion and up to 8-fold higher rates of treatment failure than patients with TB without diabetes. Patients with TB-diabetes present a delayed sputum conversion in comparison with patients with TB without diabetes. In a study from China, there was a higher proportion of patients with TB-diabetes who had positive sputum smears at two months (21.7% *vs.* 5.6%, RR 3.85, 95%CI 2.24–6.63) and who failed treatment (10.3% *vs.* 2.3%, RR 4.46, 95%CI 1.96–10.18) compared with patients with TB without diabetes [10].

Patients with diabetes have been reported to have suboptimal serum levels of rifampin, and this may be linked to poor outcomes and acquired drug resistance; this finding has been reported across different settings and ethnicities [11 - 13].

Diabetes can significantly increase the risk of developing MDR-TB. A meta-analysis that included studies from 15 countries revealed that diabetes has a significant association with MDR-TB (OR:1.97, 95%CI:1.58-2.45). This significant association persisted when adjusting for income level and type of diabetes [14]. A study from Mexico showed that patients with TB and type 2 diabetes mellitus presented a 4.7-fold (95%CI: 1.4–11.3) higher risk of developing drug resistance and a 3.5-fold (95%CI: 1.1–11.1) higher risk of developing multi-drug resistance tuberculosis [15].

The mechanisms that explain these findings have not been completely defined. Patients with poor glycemic control have modifications in their metabolism that are associated with a reduction in serum concentrations of antituberculosis drugs, especially those of rifampicin. In turn, the interaction of rifampin (and to a lesser degree ethionamide and prothionamide) with oral hypoglycemic agents at the level of cytochrome P450 results in a reduction in the activity of the latter with the consequent poor glycemic control [15].

Patients with diabetes also have an increased risk of adverse drug events. Patients with longstanding diabetes might have a renal impairment that could be aggravated by the second line injectables used for the treatment of MDR-TB. Several antituberculosis drugs (isoniazid, ethionamide/prothionamide, cyclo-serine, and linezolid) can exacerbate the neuropathy of diabetic patients [15]. Likewise, diabetes can cause gastroparesis increasing the risk of nausea and vomiting associated with ethionamide/prothionamide and PAS.

EXTRAPULMONARY TUBERCULOSIS (EPTB)

Extrapulmonary tuberculosis (EPTB) is defined as infection by *M. tuberculosis*, which affects tissues and organs other than the lungs as a result of hematogenous and lymphatic dissemination.

Risk factors for EPTB include advanced age, female gender, immunosuppression (including HIV), and chronic comorbidities (diabetes, chronic renal failure, *etc.*).

Symptoms and signs are usually non-specific, and except for miliary forms, the chest radiograph might be normal; therefore, the diagnosis of EPTB is frequently delayed with the consequent increase in morbidity and mortality.

Obtaining samples for microbiological study in EPTB is more complicated than in the case of pulmonary TB; radiology and other imaging techniques are useful in the diagnosis approach by identifying abnormalities and guiding the obtaining of biopsies. Definite diagnosis requires the identification of *M. tuberculosis* by either phenotypic or genotypic methods.

Treatment of EPTB, in general, does not differ from pulmonary TB treatment regimens. Treatment duration varies depending on the site of disease; for example, central nervous system TB requires extended therapy for one year, while tuberculous spondylitis requires nine months of treatment [16].

The World Health Organization (WHO) in their 2017 treatment guidelines recommend *"in patients with tuberculous meningitis, an initial adjuvant corticosteroid therapy with dexamethasone or prednisolone tapered over 6-8 weeks. In patients with tuberculous pericarditis, an initial adjuvant corticosteroid therapy may be used"* [17].

Other occasional indications for the use of corticosteroids in EPTB are miliary forms with respiratory failure and uveitis. The recommended dose is 1 mg/kg/day of prednisone or methylprednisolone for a month and subsequent tapering.

Some forms of EPTB may require surgery in addition to pharmacological treatment, *e.g.,* tuberculous spondylitis with neurologic compromise or pericardiectomy in patients with constrictive pericarditis.

MILIARY TUBERCULOSIS

The term miliary refers to the chest radiograph image in miliary TB, where there are small (1-2 mm) nodules disseminated through the lung parenchyma that in the histopathology analysis resemble millet seeds. The HIV/AIDS pandemic and widespread use of immunosuppressive drugs and biologicals have increased the frequency of miliary TB [18].

Miliary tuberculosis is a disseminated form of TB secondary to a massive hematogenous spread of *M. tuberculosis* to virtually all tissues and organs; it can follow primary infection, especially in children, or be the result of the reactivation of a previous latent infection. It is one of the most severe presentations of the disease, and mostly affects individuals in the extremes of age, malnourished and immunosuppressed subjects (*e.g.,* a person living with HIV) and those with chronic comorbidities like diabetes, kidney disease and recipients of solid organ transplantation [1].

Although it can affect virtually any tissue or organ, the most frequently affected are the lung, the liver, spleen, lymph nodes, meninges, bone marrow, and suprarenal glands.

Clinical presentation can be severe with acute respiratory insufficiency and septic shock or a more frequent insidious presentation with fever, shortness of breath, and malaise. Physical examination is usually negative, although the fundus examination can show choroidal nodules. Upto 50% of the patients with miliary TB have meningeal involvement. As mentioned, the chest radiograph shows small disseminated lung nodules, although, in early stages, the chest x-rays might be normal; chest CT scans are much more sensitive and can show the miliary pattern even when the chest radiograph still does not show any abnormalities.

In subacute cases, diagnosis is often delayed; spontaneous sputum smear and cultures are usually negative, with a slight increase in sensitivity of induced sputum. Most cases require the collection of samples from different locations: bronchoscopy with bronchoalveolar lavage, blood cultures (especially in patients with advanced HIV), bone marrow aspiration and biopsy of affected organs for histological analysis and culture. The characteristic histopathological pattern is that of chronic, necrotizing granulomas [19].

LYMPH NODE TUBERCULOSIS

Lymphadenitis is the most common form of EPTB, accounting for up to 40% of all EPTB. It typically affects children and young adults [20]. The most frequent location is the cervical lymph nodes, but it can also affect the supraclavicular, axillary, intrathoracic, and abdominal nodes. It usually presents as a unilateral, painless swelling of the cervical and supraclavicular lymph nodes that have a rubberish consistency. Eventually, they undergo tissue necrosis, fluctuate, ulcerate, and fistulize (a presentation that is known as scrofula). Intrathoracic lymphadenopathy, especially in young children, can compress neighboring structures, including the airways causing lobar hyperinflation or atelectasis.

Diagnosis requires fine needle aspiration (FNAB), if possible, guided by ultrasound, for microbiological, molecular (Xpert MTB/RIF), and cytological testing. The Xpert MTB/RIF has a sensitivity and specificity of 85% and 92.5%, respectively *vs.* culture as a gold standard in lymph node aspiration samples [21]. Surgical biopsy is only needed when FNAB is negative [22].

OSTEOARTICULAR TUBERCULOSIS

It is a frequent presentation of EPTB. It can affect every bone, but granulomatous spondylitis (Pott´s disease) accounts for 50% of the osteoarticular cases. The disease starts initially in the anterior aspect of the vertebral body, spreading to the disc and adjacent vertebrae. In chronic cases, vertebral TB spreads to the paravertebral soft tissues with abscess formation (psoas abscesses). It eventually involves the spinal channel with the risk of compression of the spinal cord. The most frequently affected area is the thoracolumbar region. Local and irradiated pain is the most frequent presenting symptom. Simple x-rays and CT scans are the initially recommended studies to determine the extension of the disease, but magnetic resonance (MRI) is more sensitive, primarily to assess neurological involvement.

Diagnosis requires a CT-guided biopsy for microbiological, molecular, and histopathological studies. In regions with high rates of drug-resistant tuberculosis, the histopathological diagnosis is insufficient, and microbiological or molecular studies of the biopsies for drug susceptibility testing are recommended. Besides medical treatment, some patients might require a surgical procedure to relieve spinal compression.

The most common presentations of TB arthritis are in the hip or knee. There are chronic local pain, swelling, and progressive loss of joint function. If the diagnosis is delayed, there can be the destruction of the joint with deformity and limited range of motion (Magnussen A, 2016). Fistulas are frequent in chronic cases. The culture of joint fluid can be positive in up to 80% of the cases. If cultures of joint fluid are negative, a synovial biopsy is required to establish the diagnosis [23].

GASTROINTESTINAL AND PERITONEAL TUBERCULOSIS

The entire gastrointestinal tract, from the esophagus to the anus, can be involved. Tuberculosis enteritis is acquired through different mechanisms: ingestion of contaminated milk and milk products (*e.g.,* fresh cheese) with *M. bovis*, swallowing of contaminated sputum in patients with active pulmonary tuberculosis, hematogenous spread during primary mycobacteremia or miliary disease and spread from adjacent organs. TB of the intestinal tract affects more frequently the ileocecal region. The signs and symptoms of TB enteritis are non-specific, and diagnosis is commonly established late; it is often challenging to differentiate from other inflammatory conditions that affect the gastrointestinal tract. The most common symptom is abdominal pain and malaise, fever, diaphoresis, weight loss, diarrhea, constipation, and melena might be present; in some cases, there is a palpable abdominal mass. Fistula and intestinal obstruction, (the most common complications of TB enteritis secondary to intestinal stricture or adhesions) are frequent in chronic cases [24].

Diagnosis is based on imaging studies and microbiological/molecular/histo-pathologic tests of material obtained by endoscopic biopsies.

Tuberculosis peritonitis is secondary to hematogenous dissemination or spreads from adjacent foci (intestinal or genitourinary TB). Exudative ascites is the most common finding (up to 90% of patients with peritoneal TB). Later in the course of the disease, ascites is absorbed with the development of a fibroadhesive phase of the disease.

For diagnosis, peritoneal fluid has a low yield in microbiologic and molecular tests. Some experts recommend the measurement of adenosine deaminase (ADA), and it is reported to have high sensitivity and specificity. If the analysis of peritoneal fluid is negative, CT guided, or laparoscopic biopsy would be necessary. Surgery is needed for complications such as intestinal perforation, bleeding, or bowel obstruction [24].

CENTRAL NERVOUS SYSTEM (CNS) TUBERCULOSIS

CNS tuberculosis (TB) is among the least common but more overwhelming forms of human tuberculosis. CNS TB is the result of hematogenous spread during the dissemination of the disease. It is the form of TB disease with poorer prognosis with high morbidity and mortality (up to 40%).

CNS tuberculosis infection can be categorized into three types of illness: subacute or chronic meningitis, intracranial tuberculoma, and spinal tuberculous arachnoiditis. Meningitis is the most frequent presentation of CNS TB; other presentations include cerebral tuberculomas and periarteritis with vascular thrombosis and ischemic stroke.

Meningeal TB is a chronic form of insidious meningitis that frequently is complicated by basal arachnoiditis, which leads to obstructive hydrocephalus and cranial hypertension. Initial symptoms include headache, malaise, and progressive lethargy, and coma. Due to the basal arachnoiditis, there is a compromise of cranial nerves III, IV, and VI and long nervous tracts. Intracranial tuberculoma can produce headaches, seizures, or neurological compromise [25].

MRI is the gold standard for imaging diagnosis. Hypercaptation of the meninges is highly suggestive of TB meningitis; other findings include ring-enhancing lesions and peripheral edema with areas of vascular infarction.

The analysis of cerebrospinal fluid (CSF) typically shows elevated protein levels and low glucose concentration with mononuclear pleocytosis. Smears of CSF have very low sensitivity, and culture takes several weeks for the turnaround of results. The Xpert MTB/RIF is recommended as the first test to be carried out in CSF due to it sensitivity which is reported at 79.5% (*vs.* culture) with a specificity of 98.6% and the fast turnaround of the results (2 hours) [26].

As mentioned, the duration of the antituberculosis treatment regimen should be at least one year (Table **1**), initially supported by corticosteroids. Patients with hydrocephalus require surgery for ventriculoperitoneal shunt placement.

GENITOURINARY (GU) TUBERCULOSIS

Peak incidence for urogenital TB is between the ages of 20 and 40 years, with a 2:1 ratio of men to women [27]. GU-TB is secondary to hematogenous dissemination and initially is asymptomatic. Eventually, the spread of disease to the ureter and bladder will produce lower urinary tract symptoms: dysuria, sterile pyuria, and microscopic hematuria in up to 90% of the cases. Obstructive uropathy will lead to hydronephrosis.

Imaging studies (ultrasonography, CT scans, and intravenous pyelogram) can show calcifications, ureteral strictures, and pelvis dilation. Definite diagnosis is established by the demonstration of the presence of *M. tuberculosis* in urine cultures.

The involvement of the prostate, epididymis, and testicles is common with subsequent subacute prostatitis and epididymo-orchitis. The diagnosis can be established by testing urine and prostatic fluid or through FNAB or open biopsy.

In females, bilateral involvement in the Fallopian tubes is common (up to 80%), and it is a cause of pelvic pain and infertility. Hysterosalpingography will demonstrate tube obstruction, and culture of menstrual fluid, endometrial biopsy, or of other affected tissues through laparoscopy will confirm the diagnosis [1].

LARYNGEAL TUBERCULOSIS

Laryngeal tuberculosis is usually secondary to pulmonary disease, and it is considered the most contagious form of TB. The main symptoms will be dysphonia and weight loss, but patients also can have cough, dysphagia, stridor, and hemoptysis. During laryngoscopy, laryngeal tuberculosis is characterized by the presence of nodules or ulcerations in the larynx, vocal cords, epiglottis, arytenoids, interarytenoid space, aryepiglottic fold and in the subglottic/cricoary-tenoid region; it can be misdiagnosed as laryngeal cancer.

The diagnosis can be confirmed through sputum cultures/molecular testing with identification of *M. tuberculosis*, and laryngeal biopsy for microbiologic studies and histopathology.

Most cases respond well to antituberculosis treatment with resolution of the laryngeal lesion. Occasionally patients with stridor and airway obstruction may require tracheostomy for airway management. A small proportion of the patients will report residual symptoms (dysphonia being the most common) and will require surgical treatment to resect, for example, a stenotic posterior commissure [28].

PERICARDIAL TUBERCULOSIS

It can be the result of the spread of the infection from the lung or airways, adjacent lymph nodes, osteoarticular lesions (spine, sternum, ribs), or through hematogenous seeding in patients with miliary tuberculosis. Rarely is an isolated entity [1].

Clinical manifestations of pericarditis (chest pain, cough, dyspnea, fever, malaise, weight loss) are non-specific and overlap with other diseases such as pleural tuberculosis and chronic pneumonia. Signs of cardiac failure are the result of the accumulation of fluid and cardiac tamponade or due to restrictive pericarditis. Cardiac tamponade is a clinical diagnosis characterized by jugular venous ingurgitation, hypotension, and diminished heart sounds. Echocardiography is useful to confirm the diagnosis of pericardial disease and complications such as constrictive pericarditis and cardiac tamponade and to guide the needle aspiration of pericardial fluid. An ultrasound examination will reveal an anechoic effusion and a thickened pericardium with echogenic coating and fibrin strands. It also will allow assessing the right ventricular cavity because in cases of tamponade, its diameter will be reduced, and there might be a paradoxical inward motion or even collapse of the free wall [29].

Tuberculosis pericarditis fluid is an exudate with high protein content and increased leukocyte count, predominantly mononuclear. The sensitivity of smears for the detection of acid-fast bacilli is low (<10%); culture sensitivity is also low, and some experts recommend the ADA test. If tests are negative pericardial biopsy through thoracoscopy will be needed to establish the diagnosis.

Treatment regimens recommended for pericardial TB are the same as for pulmonary TB; pericardiocentesis is a life-saving intervention in patients with cardiac tamponade [29].

PLEURAL TUBERCULOSIS

Pleural tuberculosis is the second most common form of EPTB after tuberculous lymphadenitis. In TB endemic areas, the pleural disease accounts for 20-30% of TB cases [30].

Pleural effusions were thought to be purely a hypersensitivity cell-mediated (T-helper type 1) delayed reaction due to the presence of mycobacterial antigen in the pleural space spreading from subpleural foci. However, evidence suggests that serous pleural effusions are the result of paucibacillary infections that have spread from the lung parenchyma [31]. Ipsilateral lung parenchymal infiltrates are seen in chest radiographs in 20-50%; CT scans increase sensitivity to detect parenchymal involvement in up to 80% of the cases.

Pleural TB may be a manifestation of primary TB or part of reactivation disease. In endemic regions, pleural TB is seen mostly in young individuals during the primary infection, while in low burden regions is usually a manifestation of reactivation TB in older subjects.

Typically, it is an acute illness with fever, pleuritic chest pain, nonproductive cough, dyspnea, and systemic symptoms (fever, night sweats, chills). In most cases, the effusion is unilateral of variable volume. These effusions are self-limited (even without antituberculosis treatment); however, if untreated, up to two-thirds of the patients will progress to active pulmonary tuberculosis within five years [32]. Pleural tuberculosis is more frequent in patients with HIV, who also have a higher frequency of disseminated disease at the time of diagnosis. Patients with HIV-TB co-infection have more systemic symptoms, organomegaly, and lymphadenopathy [33].

Thoracic ultrasound is now the standard of care for performing thoracentesis and closed pleural biopsies [34]. TB pleural effusions are straw color exudates with elevated levels of protein and lactic dehydrogenase (LDH) when compared with those of the serum [35]. Leucocyte cell count ranges from 1,000 to 6,000 cells/mL. Initially, there is a predominance of neutrophils, but after a couple of weeks, there is a lymphocyte predominance. Glucose levels in TB effusions range from 60 mg/dL and 100 mg/dL but can be lower than 50 mg/dL and as low as 30 mg/dL in up to 20% of the cases. Low pleural glucose and low pH (<7.20) suggest the possibility of an empyema and tube drainage should be considered [36].

Microscopy for AFB in the pleural fluid can identify *M. tuberculosis* in fewer than 10% of cases. Culture sensitivity will vary according to the type of media. Solid media cultures have very low sensitivity (10-30%), while liquid media sensitivity has been reported as high as 70% [37].

Adenosine deaminase (ADA) levels are most useful when there is a moderate to high suspicion of pleural TB. The most accurate threshold seems to be between 40 and 60 U/L [38]. There are false negatives and false-positives when interpreting the ADA levels [39]. In the early stages of TB pleural effusions, ADA results might be falsely negative. False-positive ADA results can be seen in patients with rheumatoid effusions, parapneumonic effusions, empyema with different etiology, mesothelioma, lung cancer, and hematologic malignancies [40].

If the pleural fluid analysis is non-diagnostic, the following procedure should be a pleural biopsy. The presence of caseating granulomas with or without the presence of acid-fast bacilli is highly suggestive of pleural TB. Pleural tissue can be obtained either through closed pleural needle biopsies, thoracoscopy, or open thoracotomy. Needle biopsies should be guided by ultrasound. Pleural biopsies during thoracotomy have been reported with 100% sensitivity, but due to the high yield and less invasive nature of thoracoscopy, open surgical biopsies are seldom required [36].

Chronic tuberculosis of the pleural space results in a purulent TB effusion. The empyema evolution goes through 3 stages: an exudative phase characterized by a clear, viscous fluid, a fibrinopurulent phase with purulent fluid, and an organizing phase with pachypleuritis. Empyema can result in fibrothorax in up to 50% of the patients with pachypleuritis and lung function impairment [41].

Occasionally the purulent pleural fluid will extend into the chest wall, a condition known as *empyema necessitans,* and can drain through the skin of the chest wall.

Pharmacologic treatment for pleural tuberculosis is the same as for pulmonary TB. Therapeutic thoracentesis has been associated with a rapid improvement in dyspnea. Surgical intervention may be indicated in patients with loculated effusions or empyema, and in patients with pachypleuritis and impaired pulmonary function due to lung restriction [30].

TUBERCULOSIS AND THE USE OF BIOLOGIC AGENTS AN RHEUMATOLOGY

Treatment of rheumatic diseases (RD) with non-steroidal anti-inflammatory drugs, steroids, and disease-modifying drugs has two main objectives: reduce the pain/inflammation and slow the progression of the illness [42]. However, in refractory cases, the use of biologic agents has revolutionized the natural history of these diseases. There are several monoclonal antibodies targeted at inflammatory cytokines (Table **2**).

Table 1. Antituberculosis drugs and their cerebrospinal (CSF) penetration*.

Drug	Comment
Amikacin	Variable penetration; penetrates inflamed meninges better
Amoxicillin/clavulanate	Aproximately 5% of the plasma concentration
Bedaquiline	Unknown. No data available
Clofazimine	Unknown. Limited data
Cycloserine	Concentrations approach those in serum
Delamanid	Unknown. No data available
Ethamburol	Poor penetration
Ethionamide	Concentrations approach those in serum
Imipenem/cilastatin	Good penetration. Risk of seizures in children
Isoniazid	Concentration equivalent to plasma in inflamed meninges
Levofloxacin	Concentration are 65% of that in serum
Linezolid	Concentrations are about 1/3 of those in serum (in animals)
Meropenem	Adequate CSF penetration
Moxifloxacin	Good penetration in CSF (animal models)
Para-aminosalicylate	Poor penetration in CSF
Pyrazinamide	Concentration equivalent to serum
Rifabutin	Penetrates inflamed meninges

(Table 1) cont.....

Drug	Comment
Rifampin	10-20% of serum; increases with meningeal inflammation
Rifapentine	Unknown. Nodata available
Streptomycin	Variable penetration; increases with meningeal inflammation

*modified from reference [2].

These biologics have proven efficacy in rheumatoid arthritis, psoriatic arthritis, ankylosing spondylitis, and psoriasis.

Unfortunately, one disadvantage of biologic agents is the risk of reactivation of latent tuberculosis infection (LTBI) [43]. Granulomas in the latent TB foci are composed of immune cells that prevent the activation of *M. tuberculosis*, and its maintenance is critical to avoid the reactivation of TB. Tumor Necrosis Factor (TNF) is vital for host defense against mycobacterial infection, activating the macrophages and recruiting immune cells (natural killer cells, T cells, granulocytes, *etc.*) at the infection site, with granuloma formation and containment of the infection. Anti-TNF therapy interrupts the TNF-mediated immune response and disrupts granulomas with the release of viable mycobacteria. A Cochrane review and meta-analysis reported an almost 5-fold higher risk of TB reactivation in a patient receiving therapy with biologics [44]. It is important to consider that not all biologic agents are associated with the same risk of reactivation. For example, higher rates of LTBI reactivation were reported in patients with rheumatoid arthritis receiving infliximab (rate 136 per 10^5) and adalimumab (144 per 10^5) compared with those receiving etanercept (39 per 10^5) [44].

Table 2. Biologics most commonly used in rheumatic diseases.

Target	Biologic
Tumor necrosis factor inhibitors	adalimumab etanercept infliximab certolizumab golimumab
Interleukin-6 receptor inhibitor	tocilizumab
B-cell inhibitor	rituximab
T-cell costimulation inhibitor	abatecept

All international rheumatology guidelines emphasize that this high-risk population must be screened for LTBI and receive appropriate treatment to reduce the risk of TB reactivation before starting therapy with biologics. When should biologic therapy be started after receiving treatment for LTBI will vary among the different international guidelines. If the clinical situation demands the initiation of treatment with biologics before therapy for LTBI is finished, the French guidelines recommend the administration of at least two months of LTBI treatment before the start of TNF biologic therapy [45], while the Mexican Rheumatology Guidelines recommends an interval of only three weeks from initiation of LTBI prophylaxis to treatment with anti-TNF therapy [46].

REFERENCES

[1]   Bedi RS. Management of tuberculosis in special situations. Lung India 2005; 22: 138-41.

[2]   Curry International Tuberculosis Center and California Department of Public Health. Drug-Resistant Tuberculosis: A Survival Guide for Clinicians. 3rd ed. 2016; pp. 173-93.

[3]   Yew WW, Leung CC. Antituberculosis drugs and hepatotoxicity. Respirology 2006; 11(6): 699-707. [x.].
        [http://dx.doi.org/10.1111/j.1440-1843.2006.00941.x] [PMID: 17052297]

[4]   Khilnani GC. Tuberculosis and pregnancy. Indian J Chest Dis Allied Sci 2004; 46(2): 105-11.
        [PMID: 15072325]

[5]   Laniado-Laborín R, Carrera-López K, Hernández-Pérez A. Unexpected Pregnancy during Treatment of Multidrug-resistant Tuberculosis. Turk Thorac J 2018; 19(4): 226-7.
        [http://dx.doi.org/10.5152/TurkThoracJ.2018.17062] [PMID: 30407162]

[6]   Palacios E, Dallman R, Muñoz M, *et al.* Drug-resistant tuberculosis and pregnancy: treatment outcomes of 38 cases in Lima, Peru. Clin Infect Dis 2009; 48(10): 1413-9.
        [http://dx.doi.org/10.1086/598191] [PMID: 19361302]

[7]   Lin Y, Harries AD, Kumar AMV, *et al.* Management of diabetes mellitus-tuberculosis: a guide to the essential practice. Paris, France: International Union Against Tuberculosis and Lung Disease 2019.

[8]   Dumra H. Tuberculosis in special situations: Co-morbid conditions, physiological states and contraception. Astrocyte 2017; 4: 100-7.
        [http://dx.doi.org/10.4103/astrocyte.astrocyte_64_17]

[9]   World Health Organization. Treatment of drug resistant TB in special conditions and situations. Companion handbook to the WHO guidelines for the programmatic management of drug resistant tuberculosis 2014.

[10]   Mi F, Tan S, Liang L, *et al.* Diabetes mellitus and tuberculosis: pattern of tuberculosis, two-month smear conversion and treatment outcomes in Guangzhou, China. Trop Med Int Health 2013; 18(11): 1379-85.
        [http://dx.doi.org/10.1111/tmi.12198] [PMID: 24112411]

[11]   Requena-Méndez A, Davies G, Ardrey A, *et al.* Pharmacokinetics of rifampin in Peruvian tuberculosis patients with and without comorbid diabetes or HIV. Antimicrob Agents Chemother 2012; 56(5): 2357-63.
        [http://dx.doi.org/10.1128/AAC.06059-11] [PMID: 22330931]

[12]   Medellín-Garibay SE, Cortez-Espinosa N, Milán-Segovia RC, *et al.* Clinical Pharmacokinetics of Rifampin in Patients with Tuberculosis and Type 2 Diabetes Mellitus: Association with Biochemical and Immunological Parameters. Antimicrob Agents Chemother 2015; 59(12): 7707-14.
        [http://dx.doi.org/10.1128/AAC.01067-15] [PMID: 26438503]

[13]   Nijland HMJ, Ruslami R, Stalenhoef JE, *et al.* Exposure to rifampicin is strongly reduced in patients with tuberculosis and type 2 diabetes. Clin Infect Dis 2006; 43(7): 848-54.
        [http://dx.doi.org/10.1086/507543] [PMID: 16941365]

[14]   Tegegne BS, Mengesha MM, Teferra AA, Awoke MA, Habtewold TD. Association between diabetes mellitus and multi-drug-resistant tuberculosis: evidence from a systematic review and meta-analysis. Syst Rev 2018; 7(1): 161.
[http://dx.doi.org/10.1186/s13643-018-0828-0] [PMID: 30322409]

[15]   Pérez-Navarro LM, Fuentes-Domínguez FJ, Zenteno-Cuevas R. Type 2 diabetes mellitus and its influence in the development of multidrug resistance tuberculosis in patients from southeastern Mexico. J Diabetes Complications 2015; 29(1): 77-82.
[http://dx.doi.org/10.1016/j.jdiacomp.2014.09.007] [PMID: 25303784]

[16]   Ramírez-Lapausa M, Menéndez-Saldaña A, Noguerado-Asensio A. [Extrapulmonary tuberculosis]. Rev Esp Sanid Penit 2015; 17(1): 3-11.
[http://dx.doi.org/10.4321/S1575-06202015000100002] [PMID: 25803112]

[17]   World Health Organization 2017 Guidelines for treatment of drug-susceptible tuberculosis and patient care, 2017 update ISBN 978-92-4-155000-0.

[18]   Sharma SK, Mohan A. Miliary tuberculosis. Microbiol Spectrum 2017; 5(2).
[http://dx.doi.org/10.1128/9781555819866.ch29]

[19]   Espinosa-Gimeno A, Martínez-Sanz J, Asong-Engonga L, Rodríguez-Zapata M. Protocolo diagnóstico y terapéutico de las tuberculosis extrapulmonares. Medicine (Baltimore) 2014; 11(52): 3091-7.

[20]   Peto HM, Pratt RH, Harrington TA, LoBue PA, Armstrong LR. Epidemiology of extrapulmonary tuberculosis in the United States, 1993-2006. Clin Infect Dis 2009; 49(9): 1350-7.
[http://dx.doi.org/10.1086/605559] [PMID: 19793000]

[21]   Laniado-Laborin R. Current alternatives for diagnostic confirmation of pediatric tuberculosis. Neumol Pediatr 2015; 10(4): 174-8.

[22]   Fontanilla JM, Barnes A, von Reyn CF. Current diagnosis and management of peripheral tuberculous lymphadenitis. Clin Infect Dis 2011; 53(6): 555-62.
[http://dx.doi.org/10.1093/cid/cir454] [PMID: 21865192]

[23]   Colmenero JD, Ruiz-Mesa JD, Sanjuan-Jiménez R, Sobrino B, Morata P. Establishing the diagnosis of tuberculous vertebral osteomyelitis. Eur Spine J 2013; 22 (Suppl. 4): 579-86.
[http://dx.doi.org/10.1007/s00586-012-2348-2] [PMID: 22576157]

[24]   Choi EH, Coyle WJ. Gastrointestinal tuberculosis. Microbiol Spectrum 2016; 4(6).
[http://dx.doi.org/10.1128/microbiolspec.TNMI7-0014-2016]

[25]   Leonard JM. Central nervous system tuberculosis. Microbiol Spectrum 2017; 5(2).
[http://dx.doi.org/10.1128/9781555819866.ch20]

[26]   World Health Organization . Automated real-time nucleic acid amplification technology for rapid and simultaneous detection of tuberculosis and rifampicin resistance: Xpert MTB/RIF assay for the diagnosis of pulmonary and extrapulmonary TB in adults and children. Policy update. ISBN: 978 92 4 150633 5.

[27]   Yuan J. Genitourinary presentation of tuberculosis. Rev Urol 2015; 17(2): 102-5.
[http://dx.doi.org/10.3909/riu0679] [PMID: 27222648]

[28]   Benwill JL, Sarria JC. Laryngeal tuberculosis in the United States of America: a forgotten disease. Scand J Infect Dis 2014; 46(4): 241-9.
[http://dx.doi.org/10.3109/00365548.2013.877157] [PMID: 24628484]

[29]   Heller T, Lessells RJ, Wallrauch C, Brunetti E. Tuberculosis pericarditis with cardiac tamponade: management in the resource-limited setting. Am J Trop Med Hyg 2010; 83(6): 1311-4.
[http://dx.doi.org/10.4269/ajtmh.2010.10-0271] [PMID: 21118941]

[30]   Shaw JA, Irusen EM, Diacon AH, Koegelenberg CF. Pleural tuberculosis: A concise clinical review. Clin Respir J 2018; 12(5): 1779-86.
[http://dx.doi.org/10.1111/crj.12900] [PMID: 29660258]

[31]   Ruan SY, Chuang YC, Wang JY, *et al.* Revisiting tuberculous pleurisy: pleural fluid characteristics and diagnostic yield of mycobacterial culture in an endemic area. Thorax 2012; 67(9): 822-7.
[http://dx.doi.org/10.1136/thoraxjnl-2011-201363] [PMID: 22436167]

[32]   Casalini AG, Cusmano F, Sverzellati N, Mori PA, Majori M. An undiagnosed pleural effusion with surprising consequences. Respir Med Case Rep 2017; 22: 53-6.
[http://dx.doi.org/10.1016/j.rmcr.2017.05.007] [PMID: 28702335]

[33]   Gopi A, Madhavan SM, Sharma SK, Sahn SA. Diagnosis and treatment of tuberculous pleural effusion in 2006. Chest 2007; 131(3): 880-9.
[http://dx.doi.org/10.1378/chest.06-2063] [PMID: 17356108]

[34]   Koegelenberg CF, von Groote-Bidlingmaier F, Bolliger CT. Transthoracic ultrasonography for the respiratory physician. Respiration 2012; 84(4): 337-50.
[http://dx.doi.org/10.1159/000339997] [PMID: 22832423]

[35]   Light RW, Macgregor MI, Luchsinger PC, Ball WC Jr. Pleural effusions: the diagnostic separation of transudates and exudates. Ann Intern Med 1972; 77(4): 507-13.
[http://dx.doi.org/10.7326/0003-4819-77-4-507] [PMID: 4642731]

[36]   Vorster MJ, Allwood BW, Diacon AH, Koegelenberg CFN. Tuberculous pleural effusions: advances and controversies. J Thorac Dis 2015; 7(6): 981-91.
[http://dx.doi.org/10.3978/j.issn.2072-1439.2015.02.18] [PMID: 26150911]

[37]   Maartens G, Bateman ED. Tuberculous pleural effusions: increased culture yield with bedside inoculation of pleural fluid and poor diagnostic value of adenosine deaminase. Thorax 1991; 46(2): 96-9.
[http://dx.doi.org/10.1136/thx.46.2.96] [PMID: 1901672]

[38]   Krenke R, Korczyński P. Use of pleural fluid levels of adenosine deaminase and interferon gamma in the diagnosis of tuberculous pleuritis. Curr Opin Pulm Med 2010; 16(4): 367-75.
[http://dx.doi.org/10.1097/MCP.0b013e32833a7154] [PMID: 20473171]

[39]   Laniado-Laaborin R. Adenosinedeaminase in the diagnosis of tuberculous pleural effusion: is it really an ideal test? A word of caution (Editorial). Chest 2005; 127: 417-8.
[http://dx.doi.org/10.1378/chest.1272.2.417]

[40]   Lee SJ, Kim HS, Lee SH, *et al.* Factors influencing pleural adenosine deaminase level in patients with tuberculous pleurisy. Am J Med Sci 2014; 348(5): 362-5.
[http://dx.doi.org/10.1097/MAJ.0000000000000260] [PMID: 24762755]

[41]   Candela A, Andujar J, Hernández L, *et al.* Functional sequelae of tuberculous pleurisy in patients correctly treated. Chest 2003; 123(6): 1996-2000.
[http://dx.doi.org/10.1378/chest.123.6.1996] [PMID: 12796180]

[42]   Handa R, Upadhyaya S, Kapoor S, *et al.* Tuberculosis and biologics in rheumatology: A special situation. Int J Rheum Dis 2017; 20(10): 1313-25.
[http://dx.doi.org/10.1111/1756-185X.13129] [PMID: 28730751]

[43]   Cantini F, Nannini C, Niccoli L, *et al.* Guidance for the management of patients with latent tuberculosis infection requiring biologic therapy in rheumatology and dermatology clinical practice. Autoimmun Rev 2015; 14(6): 503-9.
[http://dx.doi.org/10.1016/j.autrev.2015.01.011] [PMID: 25617816]

[44]   Singh JA, Wells GA, Christensen R, *et al.* Adverse effects of biologics: a network meta-analysis and Cochrane overview. Cochrane Database Syst Rev 2011; 16(2): CD008794.
[http://dx.doi.org/10.1002/14651858.CD008794.pub2] [PMID: 21328309]

[45]   Mariette X, Salmon D. French guidelines for diagnosis and treating latent and active tuberculosis in patients with RA treated with TNF blockers. Ann Rheum Dis 2003; 62(8): 791.
[http://dx.doi.org/10.1136/ard.62.8.791] [PMID: 12860745]

[46]   Cardiel MH, Díaz-Borjón A, Vázquez del Mercado Espinosa M, *et al.* Update of the Mexican College of Rheumatology guidelines for the pharmacologic treatment of rheumatoid arthritis. Reumatol Clin 2014; 10(4): 227-40.
[http://dx.doi.org/10.1016/j.reuma.2013.10.006] [PMID: 24333119]

CHAPTER 8

Childhood Tuberculosis

Abstract: Traditionally little attention has been paid to pediatric tuberculosis by clinicians, researchers, decision-makers, and even by national tuberculosis programs. According to the World Health Organization (WHO) Global Report for the year 2018, 10 million people developed TB in 2017, with 1 million of those being children under15 years of age. In the same year, there were 1.3 million deaths due to tuberculosis among HIV-negative people; children accounted for 15% of all deaths from TB, a percentage higher than their share of estimated cases.

Clinical presentation of pulmonary TB varies according to the age of the patient. Infants frequently will present with reduced playfulness, fever, dry cough, and dyspnea; children usually have dry cough as the only symptom, whereas in adolescents, the clinical manifestations are very similar to those of adults with fever and productive cough.

Lymphadenopathy is the most common type of extrapulmonary TB in children. The most commonly involved sites are the anterior cervical, posterior cervical triangle, submandibular, and supraclavicular lymph nodes.

BCG is the only vaccine available for clinical use in TB worldwide. Its overall efficacy for preventing tuberculosis is around 50% (range 0-80%). It is especially useful in the prevention of severe forms of the disease in children, including disseminated disease and meningeal tuberculosis. It does not prevent pulmonary tuberculosis effectively.

Keywords: BCG, Childhood, IGRA, Lymphadenopathy, Meningitis, Tuberculosis, Vaccination.

INTRODUCTION

Childhood tuberculosis always reflects recent transmission and is, therefore, a reliable indicator of the degree of control of the tuberculosis epidemic in a community. Nevertheless, traditionally little attention has been paid to pediatric tuberculosis by clinicians, researchers, decision-makers, and even by national tuberculosis programs.From an epidemiological perspective regarding the control of the disease, little interest has been paid to childhood TB since children have traditionally been considered to be non-contagious [1].

Rafael Laniado-Laborín

According to the World Health Organization (WHO) Global Report for the year 2018, 10 million people (range 9.0-11.1 million) developed TB in 2017, with 1 million of those being children <15 years of age. In the same year, there were 1.3 million deaths due to tuberculosis among HIV-negative people and 300,000 additional deaths from TB among HIV-positive people (10% of those in HIV-positive children). Children accounted for 15% of all deaths from TB, a percentage higher than their share of estimated cases; this suggests more inadequate access to diagnosis and treatment [2].

Pediatric cases account for 5% of total TB cases in developed countries and up to 25% in developing countries. Given the difficulty that exists to establish the bacteriological diagnosis of tuberculosis in children, the diagnosis in this age group has been relegated for years in the priorities of national tuberculosis programs.

CLINICAL FEATURES OF TUBERCULOSIS

Pulmonary TB

Pulmonary and thoracic lymphadenopathy is the most common clinical manifestations of pediatric tuberculosis. Most cases of tuberculosis infection are acquired by inhalation of the bacilli. Inhalation of bacilli is followed by lower lobe pneumonitis as the initial focus of infection and later by regional lymphangitis and lymphadenopathy (including hilar and mediastinal lymphadenitis). The combination of pneumonitis, lymphangitis, and adenitis was known in the older literature as a Ghon complex. After that, the infection: a) can be contained without clinical manifestations (although with the development of a positive tuberculin or IGRA test), b) can progress to pulmonary disease, c) progress to disseminated disease or d) persist as latent infection (with the risk of later reactivation).

Clinical presentation of pulmonary TB varies according to the age of the patient. Infants frequently will present with reduced playfulness, fever, dry cough, and dyspnea; children usually have dry cough as the only symptom, whereas in adolescents, the clinical manifestations are very similar to those of adults with fever and productive cough. Classic symptoms are more specific in children three years of age or older and perform poorly in HIV-infected children [3].

Chest radiography (both posteroanterior and lateral views) should be obtained in any child with a suspected diagnosis of pulmonary TB (Chapter 5: Imaging methods in tuberculosis). Findings in pediatric pulmonary disease vary widely, including normal findings, hilar adenopathy, atelectasis, military pattern, pleural effusion, and lung cavities. Computerized tomography is recommended only for complicated cases due to its higher cost and radiation exposure.

Extrapulmonary Tuberculosis

Extrapulmonary tuberculosis can affect virtually all organs and systems: pleura, pericardium, extra-thoracic lymphadenopathies, meningitis, skeletal, renal and abdominal TB, and miliary/disseminated disease.

Pleural Tuberculosis

Pleural effusions are common in children with pulmonary TB (up to one-third of the cases). In primary TB, pleural effusions develop 2-3 months after infection [4].

Although for years, it was thought that pleural disease represented a hyper sensitivity reaction without pulmonary involvement, CT chest scans clearly show subpleural pulmonary infiltration.

Effusions are more common in adolescents; as with adults, the most common symptoms are fever, fatigue, pleuritic chest pain, dry cough, and dyspnea. Physical examination reveals a substitution syndrome with decreased ipsilateral chest movement, reduced transmission of vocal vibrations, chest dullness at percussion and decreased breath sounds.

Chest x-rays reveal pleural effusion, usually unilateral; only 5% of the effusions are bilateral; other radiographic findings include areas of pneumonia and mediastinal/hilar adenopathy [4].

The analysis of the fluid will show a lymphocytic exudate with high levels of protein (>50% than those of serum), high levels of lactic dehydrogenase (>60% than those of serum), and low glucose (<70 g/dL). Adenosine deaminase (ADA) levels in pleural fluid (>40 U/L) have been used as a diagnostic test for tuberculosis effusion. However, this is an indirect test and not specific for tuberculosis effusions. In regions with low prevalence, it can lead to false-positive results [5].

Since tuberculosis effusion is a paucibacillary presentation, microscopy (acid-fast bacilli) is almost always negative, and the culture yield is only 40-60%. The Xpert MTB/RIF sensitivity for pleural fluid is also only 44% *vs*. culture [6].

The most sensitive method for diagnosis of a pleural effusion is the histo pathological, culture, or PCR examination from pleural tissue samples. The observation of caseating granulomas on parietal pleura has traditionally been considered as the gold standard for diagnosis [7] with a yield of 74% in adults [8].

Occasionally, the effusion will be an empyema, usually secondary to the rupture of a subpleural pulmonary focus. Symptoms include high-grade fever, chest pain, and dyspnea. Unlike the serious pleural effusion of primary TB, empyema fluid is usually rich in bacilli with the resultant positive results in smears and cultures.

Lymphadenitis

Extra-thoracic lymphadenopathy can be due to *M. tuberculosis* or *M. bovis* infection; the latter is frequently related to the ingestion of unpasteurized milk and milk products (*e.g.*, fresh cheese). The most common sites involved are the anterior cervical, posterior cervical triangle, submandibular, and supraclavicular lymph nodes. Nodes can be large (up to 4 cm in size), and unlike pyogenic lymphadenitis, nodes are solid, without signs of acute inflammation (redness, warmth, pain), and they frequently caseate and fistulize. Symptoms include malaise, fever, and failure to thrive. The most sensitive diagnostic method is the study of lymph node tissue; however, ultrasound-guided fine-needle aspiration has become an alternative to surgical biopsy, being less invasive and having an excellent yield. The Xpert MTB/RIF test is ideal due to the small amount of the sample; sensitivity has been reported at 85% and specificity at 92.5% *vs.* culture [3, 9].

Tuberculosis Meningitis (TM)

Tuberculosis is the most common cause of subacute meningitis in children, and it can be prevented by BCG vaccination, which is a highly cost-effective intervention against disseminated and central nervous system tuberculosis in children [10].

Almost 50% of the patients with TM are under two years of age. Initially, patients have only non-specific manifestations (fever, headaches, nausea). Later, there are cranial nerve palsies (mainly III, VI, and VI) and signs of meningeal irritation (nuchal rigidity, Kerning's, and Brudzinski's signs). Finally, patients present altered alertness and intracranial hypertension.

Chest x-rays are abnormal in almost 90% of the patients (occasionally the study will show hilar/mediastinal adenopathy or miliary disease), and more than 80% of the children have hydrocephalus and basilar meningeal enhancement on cranial CT scans.

Cerebrospinal fluid is characterized by lymphocytic pleocytosis, high protein levels, and hypoglycorrhachia. Microscopy is virtually always negative for AFB, and culture yield ranges from 30 to 70%. The Xpert MTB/RIF offers the opportunity to quickly establish the diagnosis (less than 2 hours) with an acceptable sensitivity (79.5%) and excellent specificity (98.6%) *vs.* the culture as the gold standard [9].

Skeletal TB

Skeletal TB due to hematogenous dissemination is an infrequent finding in children, and most cases are seen in adolescents. Usually, a localized disease in immunocompetent children, multiples osseous lesions are common in immunocompromised hosts.

Clinical signs include local pain, inflammation, and limited range of motion. Spondylitis (especially thoracolumbar spine), arthritis, and osteomyelitis are the most common manifestations in children. Spondylitis, the most common presentation of skeletal TB, can spread to the paraspinal muscles with abscesses formation (Pott´s disease).

Arthritis is usually monoarticular, involving weight-bearing joints, mainly the hip or knee; it is almost always due to spread from a contiguous focus of osteomyelitis.

Osteomyelitis is frequent in the skull, hands, feet, and ribs. Findings include lytic lesions, osteopenia, and periosteal reaction. Since more than 50% of bone loss occurs before plain radiographs can detect it, magnetic resonance imaging is the diagnostic test of choice; MRI can reveal bone lesions months before radiographic imaging will show abnormalities. Diagnosis will require bone biopsy for culture and histopathology [11].

Abdominal TB

This form of TB is usually the result of lymphohematogenous spread from thoracic TB; it can also be a consequence of the ingestion of infected sputum or milk products contaminated with *M. bovis*. The two most common forms of abdominal TB are enteritis and peritonitis.

TB enteritis is more frequent in adolescents as a complication of pulmonary TB with cavitation and swallowing of infected sputum. TB peritonitis is also more common in older children as a result of spread from an abdominal organ or lymph node.

Most patients have chronic abdominal pain, weight loss, abdominal distension, ascites, and a palpable mass. Clinical presentation is exceptionally varied, which results in delays in diagnosis. Complications of abdominal TB include intestinal obstruction and perforation with peritonitis.

Abdominal ultrasound can demonstrate mesenteric or retroperitoneal lymphadenopathy, ascitic fluid, and visceromegaly. Computed tomography is the preferred imaging test since it can allow for the evaluation of bowel wall thickness (more common in the ileocecal region) and the involvement of abdominal viscera [12].

Miliary/Disseminated TB

Even though miliary TB is infrequent (1-2%), it is crucial to diagnose it, given its seriousness. Most cases in children are seen in infants and children under 5 years of age, usually with some immunocompromise factors (*e.g.*, malnourishment, HIV co-infection, immunosuppressive therapy).

Due to its hematogenous dissemination, multiorgan involvement is widespread. Symptoms include fever, diaphoresis, dry cough, weight loss, anorexia, and dyspnea. The physical examination can reveal visceromegaly, lymp hadenopathies, and choroid tubercles on fundus examination. Up to 40% of the children with miliary disease will have concomitant meningitis. Chest x-rays show the typical micronodular pattern with small disseminated nodules (<2 mm); however, the sensitivity of chest radiographs can be as low as 70%. Clinical signs may precede the appearance of the micronodules in a chest radiograph; chest CAT scan is much more sensitive in the detection of the miliary pattern. Sputum examination is frequently negative (both microscopy and culture), and bronchoscopy and bronchoalveolar lavage may be necessary [4].

SCORING SYSTEMS FOR THE DIAGNOSIS OF PEDIATRIC TUBERCULOSIS

Multiple scoring systems have been developed to establish the diagnosis of pediatric pulmonary TB, where bacteriological confirmation is rarely available. Tables **1** and **2** [13, 14] show two of the most frequently used.

Table 1. Keith-Edwards score for diagnosis of pediatric tuberculosis*.

Variable	Characteristic	Points
Disease duration	<2 weeks	0
	2-4 weeks	1
	>4 weeks	3
Nutrition (% of ideal weight for age)	>80%	0
	60%-80%	1
	<60%	3
Family history of TB	No	0
	Reported by a relative	1
	Proven positive AFB	3
Clinical findings	Fever of unknown origin and/or diaphoresis	2
	Positive tuberculin test	3
	Malnutrition that does not improve after 4 weeks of treatment	3
	Lack of response to broad spectrum antibiotic treatment	2
	Non-tender lymphadenopathy	3
	Joint or bone lesions	3
	Abdominal mass or ascites	3
	Abnormal cerebrospinal fluid	3
	Vertebral lesions with kyphosis	4

≥7 points: high probability of tuberculosis.
5-6 points: probable tuberculosis; treatment could be justified.
3-4 puntos: observation must be maintained, and the studies repeated.
0-2: tuberculosis negative.
*Modified from reference [13].

Table 2. Stegen, Kaplan and Toledo score table for the diagnosis of pediatric tuberculosis*.

Parameter	Points
Bacteriologic: identification of *M. tuberculosis*	7 points
Anatomopathological: specific granuloma	4 points
Immunologic: tuberculin reaction ≥10 mm	3 points
Radiologic: pattern suggestive of TB	2 points
Clinical features: suggestive symptoms	2 points
Epidemiologic: history of contact with an active smear positive case	2 points
Diagnostic criteria 0-2 points: negative diagnosis of TB 2-4 points: possible TB, needs further study 4-6 points: suggestive of TB ≥7 points: diagnosis of TB, treatment should be started	

*Modified from reference [14].

CONGENITAL TB

Congenital TB is rare. Transmission of infection to the fetus occurs *via* hematogenous spread or by aspiration of contaminated amniotic fluid before delivery. Symptoms of pulmonary TB in a pregnant female are typical (fever, cough, malaise). However, the hesitance to obtain chest x-rays during pregnancy will usually delay the diagnosis.

Symptoms in the newborn may mimic bacterial sepsis, and the onset usually occurs 1-2 months after delivery. Congenital TB is, by definition, disseminated, with multiorgan involvement. Since the differentiation between congenital and postnatal TB is difficult, some criteria can be useful to establish the distinction [15].

1. Presence of disseminated lesions in the first week post-partum.

2. A primary hepatic complex (due to inoculation *via* the umbilical cord).

3. TB infection of the placenta or female genital tract.

4. Exclusion of postnatal transmission.

The most frequent symptoms/signs of congenital TB include labored breathing, fever, lymphadenopathy, abdominal distension with visceromegaly, and lethargy [4].

LABORATORY DIAGNOSIS

All the pediatric guidelines consider the identification of *Mycobacterium tuberculosis* from any biological specimen (sputum, bronchoalveolar or gastric aspirate, pleural fluid, urine, cerebrospinal fluid, biopsies, *etc.*) as the gold standard for the diagnosis of active tuberculosis. All guidelines emphasize that every effort should be made to achieve identification of *M. tuberculosis*, although pediatric patients are usually paucibacillary.

Older children and adolescents can often produce an adequate sputum sample, either spontaneously or after nebulization with hypertonic saline solution.

The initial bacteriological demonstration of the presence of mycobacteria is the detection of acid-fast bacilli (AFB) in a clinical specimen. However, since children are paucibacillary, the results from sputum or gastric aspirate are usually negative. Given its higher sensitivity, all specimens of a pediatric patient must be processed for culture, although isolation of *M. tuberculosis* in culture from pediatric pulmonary samples ranges only from 50 to 75%. Culture also allows the identification of species (to distinguish *M. tuberculosis* complex from non-tuberculous mycobacteria) and drug susceptibility testing. Table **3** shows the yield of the different methods for the diagnosis of tuberculosis in children [1].

Table 3. Yield of different diagnostic methods in pediatric tuberculosis.

Diagnostic Method	Yield (%)
Expectorated sputum (2 samples)	<15
Induced sputum (2 samples)	±35
Nasopharyngeal aspiration (tested with the Xpert MTB/RIF)	30
Gastric liquid aspiration (3 samples)	±40
Fine needle aspiration biopsy of peripheral lymph nodes	±80

*modified from reference [1].

A paradigmatic advance in the diagnosis of tuberculosis was the development of tests for nucleic acid amplification (NAAT) [3].

The Xpert MTB/RIF system (Cepheid™ Sunnyvale, CA) is an automated polymerase chain reaction (PCR) assay that can detect the *M. tuberculosis* complex and simultaneously the resistance to rifampicin in only two hours. Unlike the conventional nucleic acid amplification tests, the processing of the sample in this system, including nucleic acid extraction, PCR amplification, and detection, is fully integrated into a cartridge. Once the sample is added with a bactericidal reagent that liquefies the specimen, and it is loaded into the cartridge, all steps are automated and contained within the cartridge. This automation ensures a practically zero biosecurity risk and allows the test to be carried out by technical staff with minimum laboratory training at the point of contact with the patient.

The Xpert MTB/RIF uses probe technology for PCR in real-time that recognizes and reports the presence of mutations in the sequence of the rpoB gene of *M. tuberculosis* associated with rifampin resistance. The specificity of the test, demonstrated by testing various types of non-tuberculous mycobacteria, fungi, and viruses, showed that the system virtually excludes all non-tuberculous isolates [16].

A prospective study from South Africa that included 452 children (24% had HIV infection) 15 years or younger reports that 6% of the children have a positive sputum smear, 13% had a positive Xpert MTB/RIF test, and 16% had a positive *M. tuberculosis* culture. Using culture as the reference standard, MTB/RIF detected twice as many cases (75.9% *vs.* 37.9%) than smear microscopy. Also, MTB/RIF detected 61.1% of the cases with negative smear microscopy. The specificity of MTB/RIF was 98.8% (95% CI 97.6–99.9) [17].

Another prospective study (from Zambia) evaluated the accuracy of the Xpert MTB/RIF assay with gastric lavage aspirate (GLA) in 788 children. Forty-eight children (6.1%) had a positive culture. The sensitivity of the Xpert for GLA was 68.8% and specificity 99.3%. There were no significant differences detected in the assay performance when stratifying by HIV status [18].

In a meta-analysis that included 18 studies and 4,461 extrapulmonary samples tested with the Xpert, lymph node tissue or aspirate had the highest sensitivity (83.1% *vs.* culture), followed by cerebrospinal fluid (80.5% *vs.* culture) and pleural fluid (46.4% *vs.* culture); pooled specificity was 98.7% across different sample types. The percentage of children included in the studies varied from 0 to 35% [19].

This latter study included 494 pediatric samples and reported high sensitivity and specificity (86.9% and 99.7%, respectively) for the Xpert MTB/RIF in pediatric specimens [20].

The use of line-probe assays (LPA) in children (both for first and second-line drug susceptibility testing) has been recommended by the WHO based on the generalization of data from adults [21, 22].

LATENT TUBERCULOSIS INFECTION

The diagnosis of tuberculous infection constitutes a fundamental step in the diagnosis of latent and active disease in children. Latent tuberculosis infection (LTBI) is defined as *Mycobacterium tuberculosis* infection without clinical or radiographic signs of active disease. Children with LTBI are at risk of developing active TB, so the detection and treatment of LTBI is an essential component of the strategy for the control of pediatric disease (Chapter 12. Diagnosis and Treatment of Latent Tuberculosis Infection).

Most TB guidelines suggest that a tuberculin test should be considered as positive if the induration diameter is ≥10 mm in any child and ≥5 mm in high-risk children including close contacts of an active TB case, and in immunosuppressed children (*e.g.*, HIV-infected children, those receiving immunosuppressive therapy and severely malnourished children).

The risk of progression from latent tuberculosis infection to active disease is low in immunocompetent children (5-10% for life). Still, in children, under two years, this risk increases to 40-50%, with extra pulmonary manifestations or disseminated disease. In untreated HIV-infected patients, the risk of progression to active disease is 5-10% per year.

Most children who progress to active disease do so during the first year after the initial infection, and 60 to 80% of the cases are pulmonary. Extrapulmonary tuberculosis is common in children, with lymphadenopathy accounting for two out of every three cases, followed by central nervous system disease, miliary/disseminated and skeletal tuberculosis [23].

TREATMENT OF TUBERCULOSIS DISEASE

Treatment of tuberculosis has several objectives:

1. Achieve cure.

2. Prevent relapse by eradicating latent bacilli using sterilizing drugs.

3. Prevent the development of drug-resistance by utilizing a drug combination regimen and ensuring that the patient completes the treatment with the regular intake of the medications.

The main reason for therapeutic failure and the development of drug resistance is the lack of adherence to treatment, which is why all international guidelines recommend directly observed therapy (DOT) with a patient-centered approach (*i.e.*, the patient decides where to receive treatment and is not forced to go to the health unit daily for DOT).

All guidelines recommend an intensive phase for the treatment of sensitive TB with a regimen that includes 3-4 drugs for two months to prevent the emergence of drug-resistant bacilli, followed by a continuation phase for four months with fewer drugs, to eradicate latent mycobacteria.

In regions with high isoniazid resistance or HIV prevalence, a 4-drug regimen that includes isoniazid (INH), rifampin (RIF), pyrazinamide (PZA), and ethambutol (EMB) for two months is recommended, followed by four months of INH and RIF. Otherwise, the patient can be treated without ethambutol to avoid the risk of retrobulbar neuritis, an adverse effect that is difficult to monitor in small children [3]. Table **4** shows the drug and doses used in children with pansensitive tuberculosis [24].

Table 4. First-line drugs used for treatment of tuberculosis in childhood.

Drug	Daily Dosage (Maximum Dosage)	Thrice-Weekly Dosage (Maximum Dosage)
Isoniazid (INH)	10-15 mg/kg (300 mg/day)	20-30 mg/kg (900 mg/day)
Rifampin (RIF)	10-20 mg/kg (600 mg/day)	10-20 mg/kg (600 mg/day)
Ethambutol (EMB)	10-25 mg/kg (1,600 mg/day)	25 mg/kg (1,600 mg/day)
Pyrazinamide (PZA)	30-40 mg/kg (2 grams/day)	50 mg/kg/day (2 grams/day)

Most guidelines recommend more prolonged treatment for tuberculosis meningitis and osteoarticular disease with a two-month intensive phase with four drugs (INH, RIF, EMB, PZA) plus ten months of INH+RIF for a total of one year.

The WHO with the Global Alliance for TB Drug Development has developed a dispersible fixed-dose combination (FDC). The milligram per kilogram dosing of Isoniazid (H), Rifampicin (R), Pyrazinamide (Z) and Ethambutol (E) are 10, 15, 35, and 20 mg, respectively, with the FDC formulation consisting of RHZ 75/50/150 for the intensive phase treatment and RH 75/50 for the continuation phase [25]. For the treatment of drug-resistant tuberculosis in children, see Chapter 11.

ADJUNCTIVE THERAPY

Pyridoxine (Vitamin B6, 25-50 mg/d) should be administered to children with malnutrition, diabetes, and HIV to prevent peripheral neuropathy associated with isoniazid treatment.

In patients with tuberculous meningitis, the WHO recommends an initial adjuvant corticosteroid therapy with dexamethasone or prednisolone tapered over 6-8 weeks should. This is a strong recommendation based on moderate certainty in the evidence. For patients with tuberculosis pericarditis, an initial adjuvant corticosteroid therapy may be used. This is a conditional recommendation due to the very low certainty in the evidence [24]. Corticosteroid administration may reduce the extrinsic compression of airways caused by hilar lymphadenopathy [3, 26].

MONITORING DURING TREATMENT

There are several objectives during the monitoring of children under antituberculosis treatment:

1. Determine the evolution of symptoms and signs.

2. Adjust doses of medication according to weight gain.

3. Early detection and treatment of side effects and adverse drug reactions.

4. Guarantee good adherence to treatment.

During monthly visits, the following parameters should be evaluated:

1. Symptoms (fever, cough, appetite).

2. Signs (weight, regression of lymphadenopathies or visceromegaly).

3. Bacteriologic monitoring: if the diagnosis was proven before the start of treatment, bacteriologic monitoring of sputum (microscopy and culture) or gastric aspirate should be repeated after finishing the intensive phase.

4. Control of side effects and adverse reactions (see Chapter 16: Adverse drug reactions of antituberculosis treatment).

5. Early detection of drug resistance; it should be suspected if:

   a. There are known contact with a drug-resistant case or with a patient with inadequate adherence.

   b. When the child has received the treatment in an irregular manner.

   c. When the child regimen is inappropriate (in dose or type of drugs).

   d. If despite an appropriate regimen, the patient is not responding, or his/her condition is worsening.

If drug resistance is suspected, the patient should be referred immediately to a specialized drug-resistant treatment center.

Patients must be clinically evaluated at least monthly (some cases will require more frequent evaluations). It is recommended to follow all children after treatment completion every three months for the next two years.

BCG VACCINATION

BCG vaccine (Bacillus Calmette-Guerin vaccine) has almost a 100-year safety record with more than 100 million doses administered every year; It is the only vaccine available for clinical use in TB worldwide. Its overall efficacy for preventing tuberculosis is around 50% (range 0-80%). It is especially useful in the prevention of severe forms of the disease in children, including disseminated disease and meningeal tuberculosis. It does not prevent pulmonary tuberculosis effectively (efficacy 50%). BCG is not recommended in HIV-infected infants due to the high risk of disseminated BCG disease in children infected with HIV who are vaccinated at birth and who later developed AIDS. BCG is a live vaccine, and in the absence of a competent immune response in HIV-infected children, its administration can lead to disseminated BCG disease in 1% of HIV-infected infants with an all-cause mortality rate of >75%. The risk may outweigh the benefit, especially since the efficacy of BCG in HIV-infected children is unknown [1].

The World Health Organization current recommendations on BCG vaccination are:

1. To all infants living in areas where tuberculosis is highly endemic.

2. To infants and children at particular risk of exposure to tuberculosis in countries with low endemicity.

3. BCG vaccine is contraindicated in people with impaired immunity; WHO does not recommend BCG vaccination for children with symptomatic HIV infection.

BCG vaccination in infants born to mothers known to be infected with HIV should be delayed until these infants are confirmed to be HIV negative [27].

REFERENCES

[1] Hamzaoui A, Yaalaoui S, Tritar Cherif F, Slim Saidi L, Berraies A. Childhood tuberculosis: a concern of the modern world. Eur Respir Rev 2014 Sep; 23(133): 278-91.
[http://dx.doi.org/10.1183/09059180.00005314] [PMID: 25176964]

[2]   Global tuberculosis report. Geneva: World Health Organization 2018. Licence: CC BY-NC-SA 3.0 IGO.

[3]   Berti E, Galli L, Venturini E, de Martini M, Chiappini E. Tuberculosis in childhood: a systematic review of national and international guidelines. BMC Infect Dis 2014; 14 (Suppl. 1): S3.
       [http://dx.doi.org/10.1186/1471-2334-14-S1-S3] [PMID: 24564378]

[4]   Cruz AT, Starke JR. Clinical manifestations of tuberculosis in children. Paediatr Respir Rev 2007; 8(2): 107-17.
       [http://dx.doi.org/10.1016/j.prrv.2007.04.008] [PMID: 17574154]

[5]   Laniado-Laborín R. Adenosine deaminase in the diagnosis of tuberculous pleural effusion: is it really an ideal test? A word of caution. Chest 2005; 127(2): 417-8.
       [http://dx.doi.org/10.1378/chest.127.2.417] [PMID: 15705971]

[6]   World Health Organization. Automated real-time nucleic acid amplification technology for rapid and simultaneous detection of tuberculosis and rifampicin resistance: Xpert MTB/RIF assay for the diagnosis of pulmonary and extrapulmonary TB in adults and children. Policy update ISBN: 978 92 4 150633 5 WHO/HTM/TB/201316. 2011.

[7]   Porcel JM. Advances in the diagnosis of tuberculous pleuritis. Ann Transl Med 2016; 4(15): 282.
       [http://dx.doi.org/10.21037/atm.2016.07.23] [PMID: 27570776]

[8]   Ruan SY, Chuang YC, Wang JY, Lin JW, Chien JY, Huang CT. Revisiting tuberculous pleurisy: pleural fluid characteristics and diagnostic yield of mycobacterial culture in an endemic area. Thorax 2012; 67: 822-e827.
       [http://dx.doi.org/10.1136/thoraxjnl-2011-201363]

[9]   World Health Organization. Automated real-time nucleic acid amplification technology for rapid and simultaneous detection of tuberculosis and rifampicin resistance: Xpert MTB/RIF assay for the diagnosis of pulmonary and extrapulmonary TB in adults and children. Policy update World Health Organization WHO/HTM/TB/201316 ISBN: 978 92 4 150633 5. 2011.

[10]   Trunz BB, Fine P, Dye C. Effect of BCG vaccination on childhood tuberculous meningitis and miliary tuberculosis worldwide: a meta-analysis and assessment of cost-effectiveness. Lancet 2006; 367(9517): 1173-80.
       [http://dx.doi.org/10.1016/S0140-6736(06)68507-3] [PMID: 16616560]

[11]   Rasool MN. Osseous manifestations of tuberculosis in children. J Pediatr Orthop 2001; 21(6): 749-55.
       [http://dx.doi.org/10.1097/01241398-200111000-00009] [PMID: 11675548]

[12]   Tinsa F, Essaddam L, Fitouri Z, et al. Abdominal tuberculosis in children. J Pediatr Gastroenterol Nutr 2010; 50(6): 634-8.
       [http://dx.doi.org/10.1097/MPG.0b013e3181b6a57b] [PMID: 20386326]

[13]   Delgado ML, González NE. [Comparison of the predictive ability of two scoring systems for the diagnosis of tuberculosis in children]. Arch Argent Pediatr 2015; 113(6): 491-7.
       [http://dx.doi.org/10.5546/app.2015.491] [PMID: 26593793]

[14]   López-López AG, Garnica-Torrico F, Lopez-Montecinos M. Diagnóstico de tuberculosis pulmonar en pediatría. Rev Méd-Cient. Luz Vida 2012; 3: 42-7.

[15]   Cantwell MF, Shehab ZM, Costello AM, et al. Brief report: congenital tuberculosis. N Engl J Med 1994; 330(15): 1051-4.
       [http://dx.doi.org/10.1056/NEJM199404143301505] [PMID: 8127333]

[16]   Laniado-Laborin R. Alternativas actuales para la confirmación diagnóstica de tuberculosis en pacientes pediátricos. Neumol Pediatr 2015; 10(4): 174-8.

[17]   Nicol MP, Workman L, Isaacs W, et al. Accuracy of the Xpert MTB/RIF test for the diagnosis of pulmonary tuberculosis in children admitted to hospital in Cape Town, South Africa: a descriptive study. Lancet Infect Dis 2011; 11(11): 819-24.

[http://dx.doi.org/10.1016/S1473-3099(11)70167-0] [PMID: 21764384]

[18]   Bates M, O'Grady J, Maeurer M, *et al.* Assessment of the Xpert MTB/RIF assay for diagnosis of tuberculosis with gastric lavage aspirates in children in sub-Saharan Africa: a prospective descriptive study. Lancet Infect Dis 2013; 13(1): 36-42.
[http://dx.doi.org/10.1016/S1473-3099(12)70245-1] [PMID: 23134697]

[19]   Denkinger CM, Schumacher SG, Boehme CC, Dendukuri N, Pai M, Steingart KR. Xpert MTB/RIF assay for the diagnosis of extrapulmonary tuberculosis: a systematic review and meta-analysis. Eur Respir J 2014; 44(2): 435-46.
[http://dx.doi.org/10.1183/09031936.00007814] [PMID: 24696113]

[20]   Tortoli E, Russo C, Piersimoni C, *et al.* Clinical validation of Xpert MTB/RIF for the diagnosis of extrapulmonary tuberculosis. Eur Respir J 2012; 40(2): 442-7.
[http://dx.doi.org/10.1183/09031936.00176311] [PMID: 22241741]

[21]   World Health Organization. The use of molecular line probe assay for the detection of resistance to isoniazid and rifampicin: policy update . 2016. WHO/HTM/TB/2016.12. ISBN 978 92 4 151126 1.

[22]   World Health Organization. The use of molecular line probe assays for the detection of resistance to second-line anti-tuberculosis drugs Policy guidance. 2016-2. WHO/HTM/TB/2016.07. ISBN 978 92 4 151056 1.

[23]   World Health Organization. Latent tuberculosis infection: updated and consolidated guidelines for programmatic management. Geneva: World Health Organization. 2018. Licence: CC BY-NC-SA 3.0 IGO

[24]   World Health Organization. Guidelines for treatment of drug-susceptible tuberculosis and patient care Geneva: World Health Organization. 2017. Licence: CC BY-NC-SA 3.0 IGO.

[25]   World Health Organization. Statement on the use of child-friendly fixed-dose combinations for the treatment of TB in children Accessed January 17 2019. http://www.who.int/tb/areas-of-work/children

[26]   Faddoul D. Childhood Tuberculosis: An Overview. Adv Pediatr 2015; 62(1): 59-90.
[http://dx.doi.org/10.1016/j.yapd.2015.04.001] [PMID: 26205109]

[27]   World Health Organization. Safety of BCG vaccine in HIV-infected children. Wkly Epidemiol Rec 2007; 82(3): 22.

CHAPTER 9

Tuberculosis in Persons Living with HIV

Abstract: The lifetime risk of developing active TB in subjects with latent tuberculosis infection without the human immunodeficiency infection (HIV) co-infection is 5-10%; for people living with HIV (PLWHIV), the annual risk is 3-16% per year.

The interaction of these two pathogens is complex: HIV-1 co-infection is the most significant risk factor for developing active tuberculosis, while *M. tuberculosis* co-infection leads to increased viral replication and disease progression.

Clinical presentation will vary depending on the degree of immunodeficiency. Patients with higher CD4 cell counts can present with the classic symptoms, while the clinical presentation of TB in patients with advanced immunodeficiency (less than 200 cells/mm^3) is usually atypical. Extrapulmonary tuberculosis is more frequent among co-infected individuals regardless of the CD4 cell counts, occurring in up to 70% of patients with CD4 counts of ≤100 and about 30% of subjects with counts of >300 cells/mm^3.

The diagnostic approach in subjects with TB-HIV-1 co-infection is the same as that of patients without HIV infection, with the goal being the microbiologic confirmation of the diagnosis.

Antiretroviral (ART) should be started in all TB patients living with HIV regardless of their CD4 cell count. Antituberculosis treatment should be initiated first, followed by ART as soon as possible within the first 8 weeks of treatment. Unfortunately, the restoration of the immune response sometimes has an undesirable effect known as immune reconstitution inflammatory syndrome (IRIS).

Keywords: Antiretrovirals, HIV, IGRA´S, Immunodeficiency, Tuberculosis.

INTRODUCTION

The lifetime risk of developing active TB in subjects with latent tuberculosis infection without HIV co-infection is 5-10%; for people living with HIV (PLWHIV), the annual risk is 3-16% per year. The higher risk of TB reactivation occurs almost immediately after HIV-1 infection despite a normal CD4 cell count, and this risk increases with progressive immunosuppression [1].

Rafael Laniado-Laborín

Antiretroviral therapy (ART) dramatically reduces TB incidence in subjects infected with HIV-1. Still, even with ART, the risk of developing TB is higher in subjects living with HIV than in the general population [2].

The HIV-retrovirus was transmitted to humans from primates during the 20th century; *Mycobacterium tuberculosis*, on the other hand, has been a human pathogen for several millennia. The interaction of these two pathogens is complex: HIV-1 co-infection is the most significant risk factor for developing active tuberculosis, while *M. tuberculosis* co-infection leads to increased viral replication and disease progression even in the context of latent TB infection [3].

HIV co-infection will influence the clinical phenotype of tuberculosis. Individuals with HIV-co-infection but CD4 T cells counts within the normal range have tuberculosis disease like that in individuals without HIV, while individuals with low CD4 T cell counts and advanced AIDS more frequently have disseminated disease and mycobacteremia. CD4-T cells are the primary target cells for the HIV-1 virus, but HIV-1 also infects macrophages; significantly, both cells are crucial for host defense against *M. tuberculosis*, with the macrophages being their main intracellular niche. Macrophages phagocyte *M. tuberculosis* and it rapidly adapts to the intracellular environment within the phagosomes and switches from aerobic to anaerobic metabolism pathways using cholesterol as a carbon source and aspartate as a nitrogen source. Macrophages infected with *M. tuberculosis* are not able to degrade mycobacteria within the phagosomes, enabling them to escape to the cytoplasm and trigger cell death pathways with the dissemination of mycobacteria to the extracellular space and consequently the infection of other cells [4].

HIV infection generates a disruption of the cellular immune response; in tuberculosis, HIV co-infection impairs the host's ability to control *M. tuberculosis* infection through different mechanisms. Replication of the virus inside the macrophages is increased at sites infected with *M. tuberculosis*. On the other hand, the HIV infected macrophages secrete lower amounts of TNF-α, allowing mycobacterial replication. In addition, the HIV-1 virus infects and depletes CD4-T cells resulting in a decreased production of IFN-γ, TNF-α, and other cytokines [5].

CLINICAL PRESENTATION OF TB DISEASE

Tuberculosis in co-infected patients can be the result of reactivation of latent infection or from the new exogenous transmission of *M. tuberculosis*. Clinical presentation will vary depending on the degree of immunodeficiency. Patients with higher CD4 cell counts can present with the classic symptoms, while the clinical presentation of TB in patients with advanced immunodeficiency (less than 200 cells/mm^3) is usually atypical [6].

In patients with CD4 cell counts over 300 cells/mm^3, tuberculosis manifestations will be similar to that of subjects without HIV-1 co-infection: usually pulmonary disease, with high fever, diaphoresis, asthenia, weight loss, and productive cough. As the immunocompromise progresses, cavities become less frequent, and disseminated disease becomes the norm with miliary disease and bacteremia. In co-infected patients, cough is less sensitive for TB diagnosis, while fever and diaphoresis are present in the vast majority of cases. However, these symptoms are highly non-specific and can be present in other common opportunistic lung infections in PLWHIV (*e.g.*, *P. jirovecii* and fungal pneumonia) [7].

Extrapulmonary tuberculosis is particularly frequent among co-infected individuals regardless of the CD4 cell counts, occurring in up to 70% of patients with CD4 counts of ≤100 and about 30% of subjects with counts of >300 cells/mm^3 [8]. The most common presentations of extrapulmonary TB include lymphadenitis, meningitis, bone and joint, skin and soft tissues, liver, spleen, pericardial, gastrointestinal, genitourinary tract, and disseminated disease [6].

Initially, chest X-rays in patients with HIV-1/TB co-infection can be virtually normal despite positive sputum smears and cultures; if there is clinical suspicion of tuberculosis, a negative chest radiograph should not exclude the need of carrying out sputum tests for tuberculosis. In advanced cases of *Acquired Immune Deficiency Syndrome*(AIDS), the chest x-rays will show disseminated airspace infiltrates and hilar and mediastinal lymphadenopathy [8].

DIAGNOSIS OF TUBERCULOSIS IN PLWHIV

Diagnosis of Latent Tuberculosis Infection (LTBI)

There are two interferon-gamma release assays (IGRA) available for clinical use: an enzyme-linked immunosorbent assay [QuantiFERON-TB Gold In-Tube assay (QFT-IT), Cellestis, Carnegie, Australia] and an enzyme-linked immunospot assay [T-SPOT.TB assay (T-SPOT), Oxford Immunotec, Abingdon, UK]. Their use, however, has been controversial in immunocompromised individuals. A recent systematic review and meta-analysis of data on HIV infected individuals reported a pooled sensitivity and specificity of the QFT-IT assay of 69% (95%CI 50-84%) and 76% (95%CI 53-90%) respectively, with an optimal area under the curve (AUC) of 0.78 (95%CI 0.74-0.82). The pooled sensitivity and specificity for the T-SPOT assay were 89% (95%CI 66-97%) and 87% (95%CI 38-99%), respectively, with an AUC of 0.93 (95%CI 0.90-0.95). The pooled ratios of indeterminate results of the QFT-IT and T-SPOT assay were 0.07 (95%CI 0.06-0.09) and 0.19 (95%CI 0.15-0.24), respectively [9].

The use of TST (Mantoux test) using purified protein derivative (PPD) as a method of determining *Mycobacterium tuberculosis* infection can produce false-negative results in the presence of immunosuppression, such as HIV infection [10]. A recent meta-analysis [11] that included 20 studies in PLWHIV and showed a fair agreement (kappa 0.37) between the TST and the QFT-IT, makes it unclear which test is optimal to detect LTBI in PLWHIV.

Disease Diagnosis of Tuberculosis Among PLWHIV

The diagnostic approach in subjects with TB-HIV-1 co-infection is the same as that of patients without HIV infection (see Chapter 6: Laboratory diagnosis of tuberculosis), with the goal being the microbiologic confirmation of the diagnosis.

In patients with HIV-1 co-infection, especially those with advanced immuno suppression and noncavitary pulmonary disease, sputum smears are frequently negative. Cultures are much more sensitive, but turnaround time will take weeks, even with liquid media. The WHO current policy and guidance recommends (strong recommendation based on solid evidence) that the Xpert MTB/RIF be used as the initial diagnostic test in individuals suspected of having HIV-associated TB [12]. The Xpert is considerably more sensitive than sputum smears for the rapid diagnosis of TB.

Tuberculin skin test or IGRAs are not useful for the diagnostic of active disease. A positive result from either test merely indicates that the individual has been infected and does not distinguish latent from active TB; on the other hand, a negative test can represent either lack of infection or energy due to immunosuppression.

In patients with lymphadenitis, fine needle aspiration should be the initial procedure of choice, and the specimen tested initially with the Xpert MTB/RIF and also sent for microscopy and culture.

In patients with advanced AIDS with disseminated disease, blood and urine culture may be helpful to confirm the diagnosis. For cerebrospinal fluid, the initial recommended test is also the Xpert MTB/RIF [12].

A Cochrane systematic review that included 66 unique studies that evaluated 16,213 specimens for detection of extrapulmonary TB with the Xpert MTB/RIF reported a pooled Xpert sensitivity (defined by culture) that varied according to the different types of specimens (from 31% in pleural tissue to 97% in bone or joint fluid). Xpert pooled sensitivity and specificity in cerebrospinal fluid were 71.1% ($CI_{95\%}$: 60.9% to 80.4%) and 98.0% ($CI_{95\%}$: 97.0% to 98.8%). For TB meningitis, the Xpert Ultra sensitivity and specificity were 90% ($CI_{95\%}$: 55% to 100%) and 90% ($CI_{95\%}$: 83% to 95%), respectively. Xpert pooled sensitivity and specificity for pleural fluid were 50.9% ($CI_{95\%}$: 39.7% to 62.8%) and 99.2% ($CI_{95\%}$: 98.2% to 99.7%), respectively. Finally, Xpert pooled sensitivity and specificity when testing urine were 82.7% ($CI_{95\%}$: 69.6% to 91.1%) and 98.7% ($CI_{95\%}$: 94.8% to 99.7%), respectively [13].

The lateral flow-urine lipoarabinomannan assay (LF-LAM) is a point-of-care test that detects lipoarabinomannan (LAM), a lipopolysaccharide component of the mycobacterial cell wall in urine in patients with active tuberculosis. A recent Cochrane systematic review on the accuracy of the LF-LAM as a screening test for active TB in HIV-positive adults (the gold standard was the microbiological reference standard, culture or nucleic acid amplification test from samples from any disease site) reported a median pooled sensitivity and specificity of 45% ($CI_{95\%}$: 29% to 63%) and 92% ($CI_{95\%}$: 80% to 97%). In patients with a CD4 count of less than or equal to 100 cells per μL pooled sensitivity and specificity were 56% ($CI_{95\%}$: 41% to 70%) and 90% ($CI_{95\%}$: 81% to 95%). The authors concluded that LF-LAM has low sensitivity to detect TB in adults living with HIV, whether the test is used for diagnosis or screening [14].

The available tests for TB diagnosis and their advantages and disadvantages are discussed in chapter 12 [15].

TREATMENT OF TUBERCULOSIS IN PLWHIV

Integrated Therapy of TB in HIV Infected Individuals

Integrated treatment of HIV-infected individuals with TB is vital for survival, and both infections must be treated simultaneously. Early initiation of antiretroviral (ART) improves survival, while delays in the start of ART, especially in patients with low CD4 cell counts, are associated with increased mortality risk.

Current guidelines of the World Health Organization guidelines recommend that ART should be started within eight weeks of starting antituberculosis treatment and after two weeks for patients with CD4 cell counts <50 cells/mm^3 (WHO, 2017). The earlier start of ART is associated with a higher frequency of TB-associated immune reconstitution inflammatory syndrome (IRIS); however, TB-IRIS is in general, manageable, and survival benefits of early ART in this subset of patients easily outweighs the risk of TB-IRIS [16].

Since TB can progress rapidly in subjects co-infected with HIV, and this is associated with high mortality, empirical treatment should be started in patients with a high clinical suspicion of active tuberculosis. The start of treatment should immediately be followed by the collection of samples for diagnostic studies (Xpert MTB/RIF, cultures) regardless of the microscopy results, due to the low sensitivity of the sputum smears in a patient with TB-HIV co-infection.

TB treatment is similar in people with and without HIV co-infection, with comparable regimens and follow-up. However, due to the interaction between the rifamycins and some of the antiretroviral drugs, the overlapping toxicities, and the immune reconstitution syndrome, co-treatment can be challenging.

Tuberculosis treatment with first-line drugs (HREZ) is generally safe and well-tolerated and as effective in PLWHIV with pan-susceptible tuberculosis as in people without HIV infection.

In patients with drug-susceptible tuberculosis and HIV co-infection, the 6-month rifampicin-based regimen 2HRZE/4HR remains the recommended regimen. In patients with drug-susceptible pulmonary TB who are living with HIV and receiving ART during TB treatment, a 6-month standard treatment regimen is recommended over an extended treatment for eight months or more. Fixed-dose combination (FDC) tablets are recommended over separate drug formulations in the treatment of patients with drug-susceptible TB. The reduced pill burden afforded by using FDCs is especially valuable in patients with co-infection taking antiretroviral treatment and prophylactic treatment for other opportunistic infections. Thrice-weekly dosing should not be used in either the intensive or continuation phases of therapy, and daily dosing remains the recommended dosing frequency [17].

Initiation Of The Antiretroviral Treatment (ART) in TB Patients Living with HIV

ART must be started in all TB patients living with HIV regardless of their CD4 cell count. Antituberculosis treatment should be initiated first, followed by ART as soon as possible within the first eight weeks of treatment. HIV-positive patients with severe immunosuppression (*e.g.*, CD4 cell counts less than 50 cells/mm^3) should receive ART within the first two weeks of initiating TB treatment. Early initiation of ART for patients with HIV-associated TB is critical in reducing morbidity and mortality [17].

One exception is TB meningitis in people living with HIV. Immediate ART is significantly associated with more severe adverse events compared with initiation of ART two months after the start of TB treatment [18].

Immune Reconstitution Inflammatory Syndrome

Antiretroviral treatment (ART) has a positive effect on the evolution of the TB-HIV co-infection by the reduction of HIV viral load and restoration of CD4 cell numbers. Unfortunately, the restoration of the immune response sometimes has an undesirable effect known as immune reconstitution inflammatory syndrome (IRIS). This syndrome includes a short-term, sometimes severe local and systemic inflammatory response.

IRIS is reported in 18% of patients with HIV-TB after initiation of ART, and mortality from this complication is 2%. Patients with TB meningitis have a much higher risk of developing IRIS (47%), and death has been reported in up to 30% of meningeal cases.

The diagnosis of IRIS is based on the clinical scenario since there are no diagnostic tests available for this condition.

TB-IRIS is seen as a paradoxical response to ART treatment. Patients on antituberculosis treatment present clinical improvement, but after the initiation of the ART therapy, patients experience clinical deterioration with lymphadenopathy, serositis and worsening of the radiographic findings [19]. Sometimes ART unmasks undiagnosed tuberculosis; unusually severe inflammatory features characterize TB in these cases. IRIS is an exclusion diagnosis and worsening of TB due to lack of adherence to TB treatment, the acquisition of drug-resistance by *M. tuberculosis*, and the simultaneous presence of other opportunistic pathogens, must first be ruled out.

A risk factor for the development of IRIS is a very low CD4 count at the time of ART initiation and a rapid increase in CD4 counts; this will provoke an exaggerated T cell response against *M. tuberculosis* through the overproduction of inflammatory cytokines. Another risk factor for IRIS is the interval between the start of the antituberculosis treatment and the beginning of ART. In patients with very low counts of CD4 (<50 cells/μl), ART treatment should be started after two weeks of anti-TB therapy; in these patients, the risk of early mortality and other opportunistic infections outweighs the risk of IRIS. All other patients with non-meningeal TB should start ART between two and eight weeks of anti-TB therapy; as mentioned, meningeal cases have a higher risk of IRIS and ART should be started after eight weeks.

Disseminated TB increases the risk of IRIS, probably due to a much higher bacillary load, since a high bacillary load constitutes a risk factor for TB-IRIS [20].

MANAGEMENT OF IRIS

Manifestations of IRIS can be transient and self-limited; however, in some cases, the inflammatory process can be severe and fatal.

Treatment for non-severe cases of TB-IRIS includes the use of non-steroidal anti-inflammatory drugs (NSAIDs), thalidomide (due to its immunomodulatory properties) and leukotriene antagonists (*e.g.*, montelukast).

Prednisone (1.5 mg/kg/day for two weeks and then 0.75 mg/kg for another two weeks) is recommended for cases of severe IRIS; according to a clinical trial, is associated with a reduced need for hospitalization and faster resolution of symptoms compared to placebo [19]. Treatment with steroids should be used only in cases of severe IRIS since there are reports that patients with advanced HIV have an increased risk of HIV related malignancies and reactivation of herpes zoster [21].

A systematic review found similar levels of non-IRIS adverse events among patients starting early ART with all CD4 cell counts compared to delayed ART. However, overall there was a statistically significant, higher incidence of IRIS in patients who initiated ART within eight weeks when compared with delayed ART initiation across the CD4 strata and in the sub-analysis of CD4 cell count less than 50 cells/mm^3 [22].

INTERACTION BETWEEN ANTITUBERCULOSIS AND ANTIRETROVIRAL DRUGS

Rifampin and other rifamycin antibiotics have the highest sterilizing activity against latent *M. tuberculosis* among the first-line drugs, and it should be used whenever the mycobacteria strain is susceptible according to drug susceptibility testing. Rifampin is a potent inducer of both cytochrome P450 enzymes (CYP3A and VYP2B6) and phase II enzymes [23].

Unfortunately, rifampin has significant interaction with many drugs, including some of the antiretroviral drugs. Treatment of patients with tuberculosis living with HIV can include antiretroviral drugs without interaction with rifampin or substitute rifampin with rifabutin. Rifabutin is a less potent inducer of the cytochrome P450 enzymes and, if available, can substitute rifampin. Rifapentine is not recommended for TB treatment in HIV-infected patients because of significant cytochrome P450 induction, and although rifampin and rifabutin are weaker inducers of hepatic cytochrome P450, both drugs upregulate other liver enzymes and are associated with significant drug-drug interactions with several antiretroviral drugs, including all the protease inhibitors (PIs), non-nucleoside reverse transcriptase inhibitors (NNRTIs) and integrase inhibitors. The simultaneous administration of rifampin and PIs is not recommended since it is associated with a significant decrease in plasma concentrations of all PIs and poor treatment outcomes, and increasing the dose of the PIs results in unacceptable rates of toxic effects.

Rifampin has an effect on the minimal concentrations of efavirenz, an NNRTI; however, this effect does not have clinical significance and the concomitant use of a standard dose of 600 mg/day of efavirenz concomitantly with rifampin does not affect the clinical treatment outcomes [6, 16]. Raltegravir, a once a day medication [24], is significantly reduced (40%) when administered with a rifampin-containing regimen. If the rifamycin is excluded from the regimen, treatment will need to be substantially prolonged.

TREATMENT OF DRUG-RESISTANT TUBERCULOSIS

MDR and XDR-TB are treated equally in patients with and without HIV co-infection since there are no significant interactions between second-line antituberculosis drugs and ART. One exception is bedaquiline, a CYP3A substrate, whose concentrations are increased when given with a boosted PI and decreased when administered simultaneously with efavirenz. Since bedaquiline prolongs the QT interval of the electric heart cycle, frequent electrocardiogram monitoring is recommended if co-administered with ritonavir, a drug that can potentiate this effect. Nevirapine, dolutegravir, and raltegravir are compatible with bedaquiline.

SIDE EFFECTS OF TREATMENT REGIMENS FOR TB-HIV

Patients receiving antituberculosis treatment and ARV therapy must tolerate a high pill burden, and adverse effects are common; special attention must be paid to potential overlapping toxicities. Both antituberculosis and ARV drugs can cause hepatic and central nervous system toxicity, peripheral neuropathy, and skin rashes, among other side effects. With so many drugs in the regimen, identifying the drug(s) responsible for the side effect constitutes a challenge.

TREATMENT OF LATENT TUBERCULOSIS INFECTION IN PLWHIV

A recent systematic review and meta-analysis included ten clinical trials that assigned 7,619 PLWHIV to isoniazid preventive treatment (IPT) or placebo. The total duration of the IPT treatment course (300 mg of daily isoniazid) ranged from 6 to 12 months, with subsequent follow up of 12–44 months. IPT was associated with an overall 35% tuberculosis risk reduction (RR: 0.65, $CI_{95\%}$ 0.51 to 0.84). The most substantial benefit was observed in tuberculin-positive participants with a relative risk reduction of 52% (RR 0.48, $CI_{95\%}$ 0.29 to 0.82) [25].

The effectiveness of isoniazid preventive therapy in PLHIV in high burden TB regions may be limited to the period during which the isoniazid is given, and it may have suboptimal efficacy in immunocompromised individuals and will not protect against reinfection after therapy is stopped. A systematic review comparing the effectiveness of continuous isoniazid (given for at least 36 months) for the treatment of latent tuberculosis infection (LTBI) in PLHIV found that the risk of active TB was 38% lower among patients receiving continuous isoniazid compared with isoniazid regimen for 6 months (relative risk 0.62, 95%CI 0.42–0.89); and 49% lower for those with a positive tuberculin skin test (relative risk 0.51, 95%CI: 0.30–0.86). Two studies included in the meta-analysis found no evidence of an increase in adverse events in the continuous isoniazid group. In contrast, a third study found strong evidence of an increase in adverse effects. There was no evidence of increased drug resistance acquisition when continuous isoniazid was given [26].

Although LTBI treatment is effective, current regimens are limited by poor implementation and low completion rates. A randomized, open-label, noninferiority trial compared the efficacy and safety of a 1-month regimen of daily rifapentine plus isoniazid (RPH) with 9 months of isoniazid alone (H) in HIV-infected patients who were living in areas of high tuberculosis prevalence or who had evidence of latent tuberculosis infection. A total of 3,000 patients were enrolled and followed for a median of 3.3 years. The median CD4+ count was 470 cells per cubic millimeter, and half the patients were receiving antiretroviral therapy [27].

The primary endpoint (tuberculosis or death from any cause) was reported in 2% of the subjects in the RPH group and also in 2% of the subject of the H group, for an incidence rate of 0.65 per 100 person-years and 0.67 per 100 person-years, respectively (p=0.30). Serious adverse events occurred in 6% of the patients in the RPH group and 7% of those in the H group (P=0.07). The percentage of treatment completion was significantly higher in the RPH group than in the H group (97% *vs.* 90%, P<0.001) [27].

REFERENCES

[1]   Tornheim JA, Dooley KE. Tuberculosis associated with HIV infection. Microbiol Spectr 2017 Jan; 5(1).
        [http://dx.doi.org/10.1128/microbiolspec.TNMI7-0028-2016] [PMID: 28233512]

[2]   Sonnenberg P, Glynn JR, Fielding K, Murray J, Godfrey-Faussett P, Shearer S. How soon after infection with HIV does the risk of tuberculosis start to increase? A retrospective cohort study in South African gold miners. J Infect Dis 2005; 191(2): 150-8.
        [http://dx.doi.org/10.1086/426827] [PMID: 15609223]

[3]   Bell LCK, Noursadeghi M. Pathogenesis of HIV-1 and *Mycobacterium tuberculosis* co-infection. Nat Rev Microbiol 2018; 16(2): 80-90.
        [http://dx.doi.org/10.1038/nrmicro.2017.128] [PMID: 29109555]

[4]   Kabali C, Mtei L, Brooks DR, *et al.* Increased mortality associated with treated active tuberculosis in HIV-infected adults in Tanzania. Tuberculosis (Edinb) 2013; 93(4): 461-6.
        [http://dx.doi.org/10.1016/j.tube.2013.01.001] [PMID: 23523641]

[5]   Lai RPJ, Meintjes G, Wilkinson RJ. HIV-1 tuberculosis-associated immune reconstitution inflammatory syndrome. Semin Immunopathol 2016; 38(2): 185-98.
        [http://dx.doi.org/10.1007/s00281-015-0532-2] [PMID: 26423994]

[6]   Manosuthi W, Wiboonchutikul S, Sungkanuparph S. Integrated therapy for HIV and tuberculosis. AIDS Res Ther 2016; 13: 22.
        [http://dx.doi.org/10.1186/s12981-016-0106-y] [PMID: 27182275]

[7]   Cain KP, McCarthy KD, Heilig CM, *et al.* An algorithm for tuberculosis screening and diagnosis in people with HIV. N Engl J Med 2010; 362(8): 707-16.
        [http://dx.doi.org/10.1056/NEJMoa0907488] [PMID: 20181972]

[8]   Naing C, Mak JW, Maung M, Wong SF, Kassim AI. Meta-analysis: the association between HIV infection and extrapulmonary tuberculosis. Lung 2013; 191(1): 27-34.
        [http://dx.doi.org/10.1007/s00408-012-9440-6] [PMID: 23180033]

[9]   Huo ZY, Peng L. Accuracy of the interferon-γ release assay for the diagnosis of active tuberculosis among HIV-seropositive individuals: a systematic review and meta-analysis. BMC Infect Dis 2016; 16: 350.
        [http://dx.doi.org/10.1186/s12879-016-1687-8] [PMID: 27450543]

[10]   Lee YM, Park KH, Kim SM, *et al.* Risk factors for false-negative results of T-SPOT.TB and tuberculin skin test in extrapulmonary tuberculosis. Infection 2013; 41(6): 1089-95.
        [http://dx.doi.org/10.1007/s15010-013-0478-z] [PMID: 23943073]

[11]   Ayubi E, Doosti-Irani A, Sanjari Moghaddam A, Sani M, Nazarzadeh M, Mostafavi E. The clinical usefulness of tuberculin skin test *versus* interferon-gamma release assays for diagnosis of latent tuberculosis in hiv patients: a meta-analysis. PLoS One 2016; 11(9): e0161983.
        [http://dx.doi.org/10.1371/journal.pone.0161983] [PMID: 27622293]

[12]   WHO: World Health Organization. Automated real-time nucleic acid amplification technology for rapid and simultaneous detection of tuberculosis and rifampicin resistance: Xpert MTB/RIF assay for the diagnosis of pulmonary and extra-pulmonary TB in adults and children. Policy update World Health Organization 2013. ISBN: 978 92 4 150633 5.

[13]   Kohli M, Schiller I, Dendukuri N, *et al.* Xpert® MTB/RIF assay for extrapulmonary tuberculosis and rifampicin resistance. Cochrane Database Syst Rev 2018; 8(8): CD012768.
        [http://dx.doi.org/10.1002/14651858.CD012768.pub2] [PMID: 30148542]

[14]   Shah M, Hanrahan C, Wang ZY, *et al.* Lateral flow urine lipoarabinomannan assay for detecting active tuberculosis in HIV-positive adults. Cochrane Database Syst Rev 2016; (5): CD011420.
        [http://dx.doi.org/10.1002/14651858.CD011420.pub2] [PMID: 27163343]

[15]   Méndez-Samperio P. Diagnosis of tuberculosis in HIV co-infected individuals: current status, challenges and opportunities for the future. Scand J Immunol 2017; 86(2): 76-82. [http://dx.doi.org/10.1111/sji.12567] [PMID: 28513865]

[16]   Manosuthi W, Kiertiburanakul S, Sungkanuparph S, *et al.* Efavirenz 600 mg/day *versus* efavirenz 800 mg/day in HIV-infected patients with tuberculosis receiving rifampicin: 48 weeks results. AIDS 2006; 20(1): 131-2. [http://dx.doi.org/10.1097/01.aids.0000196181.18916.9b] [PMID: 16327334]

[17]   WHO World Health Organization. Guidelines for treatment of drug-susceptible tuberculosis and patient care, update. 2017. ISBN 978-92-4-155000-0.

[18]   Török ME, Ycn NT, Chau TT, *et al.* Timing of initiation of antiretroviral therapy in human immunodeficiency virus (HIV)--associated tuberculous meningitis. Clin Infect Dis 2011; 52(11): 1374-83. [http://dx.doi.org/10.1093/cid/cir230] [PMID: 21596680]

[19]   Meintjes G, Wilkinson RJ, Morroni C, *et al.* Randomized placebo-controlled trial of prednisone for paradoxical tuberculosis-associated immune reconstitution inflammatory syndrome. AIDS 2010; 24(15): 2381-90. [http://dx.doi.org/10.1097/QAD.0b013e32833dfc68] [PMID: 20808204]

[20]   Meintjes G, Lawn SD, Scano F, *et al.* International Network for the Study of HIV-associated IRIS. Tuberculosis-associated immune reconstitution inflammatory syndrome: case definitions for use in resource-limited settings. Lancet Infect Dis 2008; 8(8): 516-23. [http://dx.doi.org/10.1016/S1473-3099(08)70184-1] [PMID: 18652998]

[21]   Volkow PF, Cornejo P, Zinser JW, Ormsby CE, Reyes-Terán G. Life-threatening exacerbation of Kaposi's sarcoma after prednisone treatment for immune reconstitution inflammatory syndrome. AIDS 2008; 22(5): 663-5. [http://dx.doi.org/10.1097/QAD.0b013e3282f4f223] [PMID: 18317012]

[22]   WHO. World Health Organization 2016 Consolidated guidelines on the use of antiretroviral drugs for treating and preventing HIV infection. 2nd ed., Geneva: World Health Organization 2016.

[23]   Dooley KE, Flexner C, Andrade AS. Drug interactions involving combination antiretroviral therapy and other anti-infective agents: repercussions for resource-limited countries. J Infect Dis 2008; 198(7): 948-61. [http://dx.doi.org/10.1086/591459] [PMID: 18713054]

[24]   Deeks ED. Raltegravir once-daily tablet: a review in HIV-1 infection. Drugs 2017; 77(16): 1789-95. [http://dx.doi.org/10.1007/s40265-017-0827-9] [PMID: 29071467]

[25]   Ayele HT, Mourik MSM, Debray TPA, Bonten MJM. Isoniazid prophylactic therapy for the prevention of tuberculosis in hiv infected adults: a systematic review and meta-analysis of randomized trials. PLoS One 2015; 10(11): e0142290. [http://dx.doi.org/10.1371/journal.pone.0142290] [PMID: 26551023]

[26]   Den Boon S, Matteelli A, Ford N, Getahun H. Continuous isoniazid for the treatment of latent tuberculosis infection in people living with HIV. AIDS 2016; 30(5): 797-801. [http://dx.doi.org/10.1097/QAD.0000000000000985] [PMID: 26730567]

[27]   Swindells S, Ramchandani R, Gupta A, *et al.* BRIEF TB/A5279 Study Team. One Month of Rifapentine plus Isoniazid to Prevent HIV-Related Tuberculosis. N Engl J Med 2019; 380(11): 1001-11. [http://dx.doi.org/10.1056/NEJMoa1806808] [PMID: 30865794]

CHAPTER 10

Treatment of Tuberculosis: Susceptible Strains

Abstract: The treatment of susceptible tuberculosis has evolved in the last 70 years, from requiring the use of toxic drugs (PAS, streptomycin by parenteral route) for two years, to exclusively oral treatment, with a combination of more effective and less toxic medications for six months. The cure rate with this regimen that includes isoniazid, rifampicin, ethambutol, and pyrazinamide is higher than 90% when the patient is adherent and completes the treatment. Hence, this indicates the importance of directly observed treatment (DOT), a strategy focused on the patient.

It is essential before starting treatment with first-line drugs to demonstrate that the strain causing the condition is susceptible to isoniazid and rifampin; nowadays, these results can be available in 24-48 hours by molecular methods, avoiding the delay associated with phenotypic methods.

Although the reduction from 24 to 6 months is significant, it is still a very prolonged treatment that favors the loss of follow-up. Unfortunately, attempts to reduce the duration to four months by the addition of fluoroquinolones did not have favorable results, and the recommended length is still six months.

The most recent recommendations of the WHO include the daily administration of the drugs for six months (instead of intermittent administration during the last four months of the regimen) and the administration of the four drugs in a combined fixed dose presentation.

Keywords: DOY, Drug-susceptible, Ethambutol, Isoniazid, Pyrazinamide, Rifampin, Tuberculosis.

INTRODUCTION

The treatment of tuberculosis pursues two main objectives, to cure the individual suffering from tuberculosis and to interrupt the transmission of the disease in the community. Effective treatment of tuberculosis reduces the bacillary load facilitating healing, reduces mortality and transmission of infection to the contacts of the case, and eradicates the persistent bacilli that favor relapses and the extension of resistance.

In some cases (*e.g.*, children or very ill patients), the decision to initiate empirical treatment, even before having the results of rapid diagnostic tests, will depend on the clinical judgment and experience of the treating physician.

Since the treatment of tuberculosis requires the administration of multiple medications for several months, the patient must be involved in decision making regarding the need for supervision and other aspects of treatment. Several international agencies have emphasized the need to migrate from system-centered care (benefits the system) to patient-centered care [1 - 3].

RECOMMENDED REGIMENS FOR DRUG-SUSCEPTIBLE TB

The regimen most commonly used to treat patients with TB caused by strains without resistance-associated mutations consists of a two-month intensive phase of isoniazid (INH), rifampicin (RIF), pyrazinamide (PZA) and ethambutol (EMB) followed by a continuation phase for four months with INH and RIF (Tables **1** and **2**). It is necessary to supplement the treatment with pyridoxine (vitamin B6) in patients at risk of neuropathy due to INH: pregnant women, children, people with malnutrition, people living with HIV/AIDS, people with diabetes, alcoholics, patients with nephropathies and the elderly [4, 5].

Table 1. Recommended regimens for drug susceptible tuberculosis*.

	Intensive Phase		Continuation Phase	
Drugs	**Interval Dose (Minimum Duration)**	**Drugs**	**Interval Dose (Minimum Duration)**	**Total Doses**
INH RIF PZA EMB	7 days per week for 56 doses (8 weeks)	INH RIF	7 days per week for 126 doses (18 weeks)	182
INH RIF PZA EMB	7 days per week for 56 doses (8 weeks)	INH RIF	3 times weekly for 54 doses (18 weeks)	110

*modified from reference [5].

Table 2. Doses of first-line antituberculosis drugs*.

Drug	Population	Daily	3-Times/Week
Isoniazid	Adults Children	5 mg/kg (typically, 300 mg) 10-15 mg/kg	15 mg/kg (typically, 900 mg)

(Table 2) cont.....

Drug	Population	Daily	3-Times/Week
Rifampin	Adults Children	10 mg/kg (typically, 600 mg) 10–20 mg/kg	
Pyrazinamide	Adults Children	Weight 40-55 kg: 1000 mg 56-75: 1500 mg ≥76: 2000 mg 35 (30–40) mg/kg	
Ethambutol	Adults Children	Weight 40-55 kg: 800 mg 56-75 kg: 1200 mg ≥76: 1600 mg 20 (15–25) mg/kg	

*modified from reference [5].

About the administration of the drug, once a day dosing of all the drugs is recommended, both during the intensive phase and in the continuation phase.

The WHO, in its 2017 guideline for the treatment of drug-susceptible TB [3], included the following recommendations:

1. *"In patients with drug-susceptible pulmonary TB, 4-month fluoroquinolone containing regimens should not be used, and the 6-month rifampicin-based regimen 2HRZE/4HR remains the recommended regimen"*. Strong recommendation based on evidence of moderate certainty.
   Four different trials using 4-month fluoroquinolone-containing regimens showed higher relapse rates at 18-months follow-up compared with the standard 6-month rifampin-containing regimen, despite faster culture conversion in the fluoroquinolone groups [6 - 9]. A significant concern, based on the higher relapse rate in the fluoroquinolone groups, is the possibility of increased resistance to these drugs.

2. *"The use of fixed-dose combination (FDC) tablets is recommended over separate drug formulations in the treatment of patients with drug-susceptible TB."* Conditional recommendation due to the low certainty of the evidence.
   A recent systematic review and meta-analysis and a Cochrane review showed that treatment with FDC was not inferior to separate drug formulations in terms of treatment failure, death, treatment adherence, and adverse events [10, 11]. As expected, patient satisfaction was higher among people who were treated with FDCs. Also, FDCs can provide benefits to national TB programs by simplifying the ordering, supply, and distribution of drugs. Nonetheless, WHO recommends that programs should have a stock of separate drug formulations for patients with adverse drug reactions, preventive therapy, or drug resistance.

3. *"In all patients with drug-susceptible pulmonary TB, the use of thrice-weekly dosing is not recommended in both the intensive and continuation phases of therapy, and daily dosing remains the recommended dosing frequency."* This is also a conditional recommendation due to the very low certainty of the evidence.
   Thrice-weekly dosing throughout treatment *vs.* daily dosing is associated with a higher risk of treatment failure, relapse, and acquired drug resistance; when thrice-weekly dosing during the continuation phase is compared to daily dosing, thrice-weekly dosing is associated with a higher failure and relapse rates. Thrice-weekly dosing should never be used during the intensive phase, and if used during the continuation phase, it should always be under strict direct observation [3].

4. *"In patients with drug-susceptible pulmonary TB who are living with HIV and receiving antiretroviral therapy during TB treatment, a 6-month standard treatment regimen is recommended over an extended treatment for eight months or more"*. This is a conditional recommendation due to the very low certainty of the evidence [3].

5. *"In patients who require TB retreatment, the category II regimen should no longer be prescribed, and drug-susceptibility testing should be conducted to inform the choice of a treatment regimen."* Due to the lack of evidence (there are no randomized clinical trials), the low cure rate reported with category II regimen (68%) and the risk of extending resistance in patients with undetected resistance to isoniazid [12], this is a good practice statement by the WHO.

TREATMENT IMPLEMENTATION AND PATIENT CARE AND SUPPORT

In its 2017 treatment guidelines, the WHO suggests the following TB treatment administration options [3]:

1. Community or home-based directly observed therapy (DOT). This option is recommended over health facility-based DOT or unsupervised treatment.

2. The treatment administered by health care workers or trained community providers is recommended over DOT administered by family members or unsupervised treatment.

3. Video observed treatment (VOT) might replace DOT when the technology is available.

For patient care support, the WHO also recommends staff education and training, patient health education and counseling, tracers (home visits or telephone/digital communications) treatment adherence interventions (*e.g.*, meals, food baskets, food or food vouchers, transport support, living allowance, housing incentives, or financial bonus), psychological support and treatment administration options (see above).

RECOMMENDED BASELINE AND FOLLOW-UP EVALUATIONS

Patients need to be evaluated clinically on a monthly basis for monitoring of weight (adjust medication dose if required), treatment adherence (from DOT reports), the evolution of the symptoms (fatigue, fever, night sweats, cough, sputum production, appetite, *etc*.), to inquire about potential drug side effects and adverse reactions (nausea, arthralgias, vomiting, neuropathy, jaundice, choluria, skin rash, *etc*.). During the physical examination, it is necessary to test for visual acuity with the Snellen chart and for color discrimination with the Ishihara plates.

Sputum smear and culture samples must be obtained monthly until two consecutive specimens with negative culture are obtained. The duration of the intensive phase will depend on the bacteriological conversion at the end of the second month of treatment. The presence of positive culture at the end of the intensive phase correlates with relapse after the end of the treatment [13, 14]. The presence of lung cavitation on the initial chest radiograph is a risk factor for relapse; patients treated with the 6-month regimen who possess both a lung cavity and a positive culture at the end of the intensive phase have a relapse rate of 20% (*vs.* 2% for patients with neither risk factor) [13]. It is necessary to obtain a baseline chest radiograph in all patients undergoing treatment; obtaining a chest radiograph at the end of treatment is optional.

All patients with confirmed tuberculosis should be tested for HIV, HIV RNA load and CD4 lymphocyte count in seropositive patients.

The liver function test (ALT, AST, and bilirubin) should be obtained at baseline and if the patient develops symptoms suggestive of liver toxicity. Monthly liver function tests are recommended in subjects with a high risk of drug-induced toxicity (chronic alcohol consumption, intravenous drug consumption, viral hepatitis B or C, HIV/AIDS, *etc*).

Patients with risk factors for hepatitis B or C (intravenous drug consumption, HIH/AIDS) should be tested for these viruses.

Individuals with risk factors for diabetes (obesity, family history, ethnicity) should be tested for diabetes (fasting glucose and hemoglobin A1c).

WHO SHOULD RECEIVE TREATMENT FOR MORE THAN SIX MONTHS?

The 2016 guidelines from the American Thoracic Society/Center for Disease Control and Prevention/Infectious Diseases Society of America [5] recommend that patients with cavitation at baseline and positive culture at the end of the 2-month intensive phase should receive a 3-month extension of the continuation phase with INH and RIF (expert opinion) for a total of 9 months of treatment.

MANAGEMENT OF TREATMENT INTERRUPTION

Lost to follow-up is one of the leading global problems in the treatment of tuberculosis. The clinician in charge of the case must decide when the patient returns after the interruption, whether to restart treatment all over again or continue to finish the original regimen. Discontinuation of treatment during the intensive phase has a more significant impact, and the longer the interruption, the greater the need to restart therapy from the beginning. Table **3** shows some recommendations for resuming treatment.

Table 3. Management of treatment interruption (expert opinion).

Phase of Interruption	Details of Interruption	Recommendation
Intensive phase	Lapse is <14 d in duration	Continue treatment to complete planned total number of doses (if all doses are completed within 3 months)
	Lapse is ≥14 d in duration	Restart treatment from the beginning
Continuation phase	Received ≥80% of doses and sputum was AFB smear positive on initial testing	Continue therapy until all doses are completed
	Received <80% of doses and accumulative lapse is <3 months in duration	Continue therapy until all doses are completed (full course), unless consecutive lapse is >2 months
	Received <80% of doses and lapse is ≥3 months in duration	Restart therapy from the beginning, new intensive and continuation phases

TREATMENT OF CULTURE-NEGATIVE TUBERCULOSIS

Occasionally, patients with clinical and radiographic findings suggestive of tuberculosis have negative smears/cultures and molecular tests for *M. tuberculosis*. This does not necessarily exclude active disease since there are several reasons why a patient with active TB might have negative microbiological results: recent treatment with antibiotics that have antimycobacterial activity (*e.g.*, fluoroquinolones), paucibacillary tuberculosis, saliva samples instead of sputum, excessive decontamination of samples for culture or contaminated cultures.

An alternative diagnosis must be ruled out (*e.g.*, mycosis), and all possible efforts must be made to obtain an adequate sample of bronchial secretions (induced sputum, bronchoalveolar lavage/biopsy) before accepting the diagnosis of negative culture tuberculosis.

Once the diagnosis of tuberculosis is established based on the clinical findings, treatment is started with first-line drugs (INH, RIF, EMB, and PZA) with the same regimen utilized in bacteriologically proven cases. If during treatment, cultures are eventually reported as positive with MTB, the patient should complete the full, standard 6-month regimen. Patients with negative cultures should be closely followed; if the patient presents clinical/radiographic improvement, and an alternative diagnosis is not identified, the patient must continue with the antituberculosis treatment.

The optimal duration of treatment of patients with a clinical diagnosis has not been established. In adults, there are a couple of studies that have shown good results with a 4-month regimen (instead of six months) and without a significant difference in the relapse rate when compared to the standard six-month regimen [15]. Patients will start with a 4-drug regimen, and if at the end of the second month there is a clinical improvement (and the tests continue to be negative for MTB), the continuation phase could be stopped after 2 months for a total of four months of treatment.

The clinical and radiographic evolution should be evaluated at the end of the 4th month of treatment to determine if it is convenient to extend the treatment to six months.

INADEQUATE TREATMENT RESPONSE AND TREATMENT FAILURE

Between 90-95% of the patients with ***drug-susceptible*** tuberculosis, culture will be negative after three months of treatment with first-line drugs. At the same time, most patients will experience clinical improvement (become afebrile, with reduced cough and sputum production, and experience weight gain). Patients with torpid clinical evolution or positive cultures after three months of treatment must be carefully evaluated to determine the cause.

In patients under unsupervised treatment, poor adherence must be ruled out since it is a frequent cause of suboptimal response to treatment. In patients under a DOT regimen, it should be verified that the DOT provider is effectively supervising the taking of the medicines (he/she can be delivering the medications daily to the patient without overseeing the intake of the drugs). Another reason for an inadequate response is malabsorption of the antituberculosis medications due to diarrhea, diabetes, AIDS, or the simultaneous ingestion of other drugs that interfere with their absorption.

The ATS/CDC/IDSA defines treatment failure as continuously or recurrently positive cultures after four months of treatment in a patient receiving appropriate chemotherapy. The WHO defines treatment failure as a case of TB whose sputum smear or culture is positive at month 5 or later during treatment [5, 16, 17]. For patients who meet the criteria for treatment failure, sputum specimens must be processed for culture/drug susceptibility testing and molecular tests for drug resistance to first and second-line drugs; the patient should be immediately referred to a specialty center for drug-resistant tuberculosis [18].

REFERENCES

[1]   Hopewell PC, Pai M, Maher D, Uplekar M, Raviglione MC. International standards for tuberculosis care. Lancet Infect Dis 2006; 6(11): 710-25.
        [http://dx.doi.org/10.1016/S1473-3099(06)70628-4] [PMID: 17067920]

[2]   Migliori GB, Zellweger JP, Abubakar I, *et al.* European union standards for tuberculosis care. Eur Respir J 2012; 39(4): 807-19.
        [http://dx.doi.org/10.1183/09031936.00203811] [PMID: 22467723]

[3]   WHO. Guidelines for treatment of drug-susceptible tuberculosis and patient care, 2017 update. Geneva: World Health Organization. 2017. Licence: CC BY-NC-SA 3.0 IGO.

[4]   Dela Cruz CS, Lyons PG, Pasnick S, *et al.* Treatment of drug-susceptible tuberculosis. Ann Am Thorac Soc 2016; 13(11): 2060-3.
        [http://dx.doi.org/10.1513/AnnalsATS.201607-567CME] [PMID: 27831799]

[5]   Nahid P, Dorman SE, Alipanah N, *et al.* Official american thoracic society/centers for disease control and prevention/infectious diseases society of america clinical practice guidelines: treatment of drug-susceptible tuberculosis. Clin Infect Dis 2016; 63(7): e147-95.
        [http://dx.doi.org/10.1093/cid/ciw376.]

[6]   Gillespie SH, Crook AM, McHugh TD, *et al.* Four-month moxifloxacin-based regimens for drug-sensitive tuberculosis. N Engl J Med 2014; 371(17): 1577-87.
        [http://dx.doi.org/10.1056/NEJMoa1407426] [PMID: 25196020]

[7]   Merle CS, Fielding K, Sow OB, *et al.* A four-month gatifloxacin-containing regimen for treating tuberculosis. N Engl J Med 2014; 371(17): 1588-98.
        [http://dx.doi.org/10.1056/NEJMoa1315817] [PMID: 25337748]

[8]   Jindani A, Harrison TS, Nunn AJ, *et al.* High-dose rifapentine with moxifloxacin for pulmonary tuberculosis. N Engl J Med 2014; 371(17): 1599-608.
[http://dx.doi.org/10.1056/NEJMoa1314210] [PMID: 25337749]

[9]   Jawahar MS, Banurekha VV, Paramasivan CN, *et al.* Randomized clinical trial of thrice-weekly 4-month moxifloxacin or gatifloxacin containing regimens in the treatment of new sputum positive pulmonary tuberculosis patients. PLoS One 2013; 8(7): e67030.
[http://dx.doi.org/10.1371/journal.pone.0067030] [PMID: 23843980]

[10]   Albanna AS, Smith BM, Cowan D, Menzies D. Fixed-dose combination antituberculosis therapy: a systematic review and meta-analysis. Eur Respir J 2013; 42(3): 721-32.
[http://dx.doi.org/10.1183/09031936.00180612] [PMID: 23314904]

[11]   Gallardo CR, Rigau Comas D, Valderrama Rodríguez A, *et al.* Fixed-dose combinations of drugs *versus* single-drug formulations for treating pulmonary tuberculosis. Cochrane Database Syst Rev 2016; (5): CD009913.
[http://dx.doi.org/10.1002/14651858.CD009913.pub2] [PMID: 27186634]

[12]   Gegia M, Winters N, Benedetti A, van Soolingen D, Menzies D. Treatment of isoniazid-resistant tuberculosis with first-line drugs: a systematic review and meta-analysis. Lancet Infect Dis 2016; S1473-3099(16): 30407-8.
[http://dx.doi.org/10.1016/S1473-3099(16)30407-8.]

[13]   Jo KW, Yoo JW, Hong Y, *et al.* Risk factors for 1-year relapse of pulmonary tuberculosis treated with a 6-month daily regimen. Respir Med 2014; 108(4): 654-9.
[http://dx.doi.org/10.1016/j.rmed.2014.01.010] [PMID: 24518046]

[14]   Horne DJ, Royce SE, Gooze L, *et al.* Sputum monitoring during tuberculosis treatment for predicting outcome: systematic review and meta-analysis. Lancet Infect Dis 2010; 10(6): 387-94.
[http://dx.doi.org/10.1016/S1473-3099(10)70071-2] [PMID: 20510279]

[15]   Dutt AK, Moers D, Stead WW. Smear- and culture-negative pulmonary tuberculosis: four-month short-course chemotherapy. Am Rev Respir Dis 1989; 139(4): 867-70.
[http://dx.doi.org/10.1164/ajrccm/139.4.867] [PMID: 2930066]

[16]   World Health Organization. Definitions and reporting framework for tuberculosis – 2013 revision. 2013. WHO/HTM/TB/2013.2. ISBN 978 92 4 150534 5.

[17]   WHO policy on collaborative TB/HIV activities. Guidelines for national programmes and other stakeholders 2012. (Document WHO/HTM/TB/20121) Geneva: World Health Organization 2012.

[18]   Laniado-Laborín R. Drug Resistant Tuberculosis. Practical guide for clinical management, Chapter 5 . 1ᵗed. Bentham e-books 2015; pp. 22-9. ISBN 978-1-68108-067-3.
[http://dx.doi.org/10.2174/97816810806661150101]

CHAPTER 11

Treatment of Drug-Resistant Tuberculosis

Abstract: The presence of drug resistance should always be suspected when there are risk factors for it and must be confirmed by bacteriological or molecular tests for standardized drug sensitivity. Any regimen for drug-resistant TB is more likely to be effective if its composition is based on information from reliable drug susceptibility testing.

The presence of drug-resistant tuberculosis should be suspected in patients who are failing treatment, in patients with TB relapse, in subjects coming from regions with a high prevalence of MDR-TB, and in contacts of known cases of MDR-TB. Although there are multiple reasons why treatment may fail, the most frequent is the lack of adherence to the regimen.

The most common causes of relapse include lack of adherence to treatment with the development of acquired drug resistance, treatment with an inadequate therapeutic regimen, malabsorption of drugs, and exogenous reinfection with a different strain of *M. tuberculosis*.

In patients with confirmed rifampicin-susceptible and isoniazid-resistant tuberculosis, treatment with rifampicin, ethambutol, pyrazinamide, and levofloxacin is recommended for a duration of 6 months.

One general WHO recommendation is that all patients with rifampin-resistant TB (even those with monoresistance to rifampin) should be treated with an MDR-TB drug regimen. There are three options for the treatment of RR/MDR/XDR TB. Two are recommendations for programmatic management (the short and longer regimens) and one for operational research (the BPaL regimen).

Keywords: BPaL, Drug-resistant tuberculosis, Longer regimen, Short-course regimen, Treatment.

INTRODUCTION

The presence of drug resistance should always be suspected when there are risk factors for it and must be confirmed by bacteriological or molecular tests for standardized drug sensitivity. Because the treatment of a drug-resistant case will depend heavily on the results of drug susceptibility tests, a maximum effort should be made to isolate *M. tuberculosis* [1].

The presence of drug-resistant tuberculosis should be suspected in patients who are failing treatment (*e.g.*, the persistence of viable germs in cultures after 4 months of strictly supervised treatment, or presenting positive cultures again after having converted their cultures to negative during treatment), patients with TB relapse, in subjects migrating from regions with a high prevalence of MDR-TB, and in contacts of known cases of MDR-TB. Clinical suspicion of MDR-TB will allow earlier diagnosis and initiation of the treatment (with a better prognosis for the case) and will reduce the transmission of resistant strains in the community.

In fact, the lack of improvement in the symptoms and the persistence of positive microscopy should make the clinician suspect the possibility of drug-resistant TB, and order (if it has not been done yet) phenotypic or genotypic drug susceptibility testing (DST). There are multiple reasons why the treatment may fail, the most frequent being the lack of adherence to the regimen, the acquisition of resistance during the treatment (usually due to lack of adherence or an inadequate regimen), or intestinal malabsorption.

Faced with a patient who is failing, the clinician must determine if cultures and DST were carried out and if drug resistance was present before the initial treatment. Treatment should be stopped, and a new sputum sample should be obtained for rapid molecular tests (Xpert, LPAs), culture and DST that will confirm if there is resistance to drugs, or if it already existed before the initiation of therapy if it now has acquired resistance to other drugs in the regimen [1].

When a patient presents a bacteriological relapse (history of been successfully treated and discharged as cured with negative cultures at the end of the treatment) and presents again with clinical evidence of disease and positive cultures for *M. tuberculosis*, the possibility of drug-resistant TB is highly probable since the history of previous treatment is one of the most important risk factors for this complication. This is especially frequent in patients who have been treated with unsupervised regimens. Patients treated with directly observed therapy (DOT) have a much lower risk of developing drug-resistance during the treatment. The most common causes of relapse include lack of adherence to treatment with the development of acquired resistance, treatment with an inadequate therapeutic regimen, malabsorption of drugs, and exogenous reinfection with a different strain of *M. tuberculosis*. An exception is patients with an initial pan-susceptible strain treated under DOT with first-line drugs; there is a high probability that the relapse, in this case, is due to the same pan-susceptible strain (from reactivation of latent bacilli that were not killed during the treatment). Under these conditions, it is recommended to start the primary regimen again while the DST report is available. If, on the contrary, the treatment was not supervised or was irregular, it is recommended to start with an expanded regimen while the DST are being reported, especially if the patient is immunocompromised, has a central nervous system condition or is severely ill. By expanded regimen is meant adding 2 to 3 new drugs (that the patient has never received) to the standard 4-drug regimen [1].

TREATMENT OF DRUG-RESISTANT TUBERCULOSIS

Mono-resitance Resistance to Isoniazid

In its 2019 consolidated guidelines on drug-resistant tuberculosis treatment [2], the WHO published the following recommendations for the treatment of isoniazid-resistant tuberculosis:

1. In patients with confirmed rifampicin-susceptible and isoniazid-resistant tuberculosis, treatment with rifampicin, ethambutol, pyrazinamide, and levofloxacin is recommended for a duration of 6 months.

2. In patients with confirmed rifampicin-susceptible and isoniazid-resistant tuberculosis, it is not recommended to add streptomycin or other injectable agents to the treatment regimen.

Evidence shows that there is no statistically significant difference in the treatment outcomes of patients receiving six months of the four-drug regimen and those receiving more than six months of the same regimen. This statement only applies to treatment with a daily regimen for six months. Levofloxacin is recommended over moxifloxacin due to its lower toxicity and cost. The six-month regimen is also recommended for persons living with HIV.

In patients with isoniazid-resistant TB, treatment success rates were higher when fluoroquinolones (FQs) were added to the primary regimen drugs (rifampin-ethambutol-pyrazinamide, REZ) as compared to patients treated with six or more months of the same regimen without the addition of FQs (aOR, 2.8; 95% CL 1.1–7.3); also, with the addition of FQs in patients receiving REZ, the number of deaths was reduced (aOR, 0.4; 95% CL 0.2–1.1). Finally, the acquisition of additional resistance with progression to MDR-TB was also reduced when fluoroquinolones were added to a ≥6REZ regimen (aOR, 0.10; 95% CL 0.01–1.2) [2].

Even though there is no clear evidence that including isoniazid in the regimen adds any benefit to this regimen, the fixed-dose combination tablets (that include H) may be more convenient for the patient and the TB program than the use of single drugs.

However, the recommendation of adding an FQ assumes that patients with H-resistant TB are identified before starting any treatment. In programmatic conditions, patients are diagnosed with sputum microscopy as the only test and will be treated empirically with first-line drugs. The use of the Xpert MTB/RIF as the initial test for subjects with suspicion of TB is increasing globally, but frequently will be the only drug susceptibility test performed, and resistance to isoniazid will go undetected. Finally, in some cases, the patient will be started on first-line drugs based on the results of sputum microscopy, and results from cultures will be available only after 1-4 months, depending on the type of culture (liquid *vs.* solid media culture). A large meta-analysis by Menzies *et al.* showed that when patients with mono-resistance to H are treated only with the standardized regimen of first-line drugs, treatment failure rates range from 18% - 44%. The same meta-analysis found an increment of acquired drug resistance of 5.1 times in patients with INH-resistant disease *vs.* those with a drug-susceptible disease (95%CI 2.3 - 11.0) [3, 4].

If resistance to isoniazid is detected after the results of culture are available, the guidelines recommend adding a fluoroquinolone to the regimen once rifampin resistance has been excluded.

The duration of an H-resistant regimen is determined by the need to complete six months of a levofloxacin-containing regimen. If the diagnosis of H-resistance is made after the treatment has already started, the patient may need more than six months of treatment with first-line drugs. When H-resistance is reported late into therapy with the 2HRZE/4HR regimen, a decision will be made by the clinician to add (or not) at that point an FQ and prolong the (H)RZE regimen for six more months, based on an assessment of the clinical and bacteriological condition of the patient.

In patients with extensive disease (bilateral, cavitary disease) and/or persistence of positive sputum (microscopy or culture) beyond three months, the prolongation of the 6(H)REZ–FQ regimen to more than six months could be considered on an individual basis [5].

Isolated Resistance to Ethambutol (EMB), Pyrazinamide (PZA), or Streptomycin (SM)

Isolated resistance to EMB or SM will have little impact on the efficacy of the treatment regimen. Resistance to EMB or SM will not decrease the effectiveness of the regimen or its duration. In cases with resistance to pyrazinamide, it is recommended to prolong the continuation phase of the treatment (with INH-RIF) for three months for a total of 9 months of therapy. Most PZA mono-resistant isolates are due to *Mycobacterium bovis* [5].

Poly-Resistant *M. Tuberculosis*

Tuberculosis due to organisms resistant to more than one anti-TB drug (that are not simultaneously INH and RIF) is classified as poly-resistant TB. There are many combinations of resistance, but the outcome of treatment is usually good. Table **1** shows the cross resistance pattern for the different antituberculosis drugs. Table **2** shows the recommended regimens for poly-resistant tuberculosis.

Table 1. Cross resistance for anti-tuberculosis drugs*.

Drug	Cross-Resistance	Comments
Isoniazid	Ethionamide	Very common when there is low-level resistance to isoniazid due to a mutation in *inhA* or the promoter region
Rifampin	Rifamycins	Is very frequent. Cross-resistance between rifampin and rifabutin is >80%
Ethambutol	None	
Pyrazinamide	None	
Streptomycin	Kanamycin	Not frequent
Amikacin	Kanamycin	High likelihood since it is associated to the same *rrs* mutation
Fluoro quinolones	Other fluoroquinolones	In general there is a complete class effect cross-resistance *in vitro*. However, moxifloxacin may continue to have some activity despite *in vitro* resistance to levofloxacin
Cycloserine	None	
PAS	None	
Ethionamide	Isoniazid	Very common when there is low-level resistance to isoniazid due to a mutation in *inhA* or the promoter region
Clofazimine	Bedaquiline	Cross-resistance in both directions through efflux-based resistance
Linezolid	None	
Bedaquiline	Clofazimine	Cross-resistance in both directions through efflux-based resistance
Delamanid	Pretomanid	Nonsynonymous mutation within the *fbiA* gene

*modified from refrence [2].

TREATMENT OF MDR/XDR TUBERCULOSIS

The World Health Organization (WHO) has issued for years guidelines for the programmatic management of MDR-TB, and their recommendations have been implemented in many regions worldwide [6]. One general WHO recommendation is that all patients with rifampin-resistant TB (even in cases with monoresistance to rifampin) should be treated with an MDR-TB drug regimen.

Rifampicin-resistant TB *(RR-TB)* is the disease caused by MTB strains that are resistant to rifampicin on the basis of the molecular or phenotypic DST. Rifampicin-resistant TB strains may be susceptible to isoniazid, or resistant also to isoniazid (*i.e.*, MDR-TB), or resistant to other first-line TB medicines besides rifampin (poly-resistant) or resistant to rifampin, isoniazid plus fluoroquinolones and second-line injectables (*e.g.*, XDR-TB); it can be treated either with a longer treatment (longer MDR-TB regimens) or an all oral short-course treatment.

A *shorter MDR-TB regimen* refers to a course of treatment for MDR/RR-TB lasting less than 12 months and is generally standardized. *Longer MDR-TB regimens* are treatments for MDR/RR-TB or XDR-TB, which last 18 months or more and designed using priority grouping (A, B, C groups) of second-line medicines.

Given the availability of new effective oral drugs like bedaquiline and delamanid and the significant reduction in the prices of other effective drugs like moxifloxacin and linezolid, the WHO considered that it was necessary to review the regimen composition for the longer MDR-TB regimen, and with this purpose, made a public call for individual MDR/RR-TB patient data. A meta-analysis of this data allowed the study of useful correlates of the outcome, including regimen composition. Results were recently published [7] and were used to develop the current guidelines for MDR/RR-TB treatment. To analyze treatment success, failure, relapse, and death, the 2018 IPD-MA included 13,104 individual patients' records (from 53 studies in 40 countries). To determine adverse effects (AE) that resulted in permanent discontinuation of an individual drug in longer regimens, a subset of 5,450 records (from 17 studies) supplemented with information from 10 additional studies that only reported AE from either bedaquiline, linezolid or carbapenems, was analyzed (Table **4**).

The meta-analysis showed that the fluoroquinolones (levofloxacin/moxifloxacin), bedaquiline and linezolid were the three most effective drugs, with a reduction in the risk of failure/relapse *vs.* the success of 70%, and a reduction of risk of death *vs.* the success of 80% (Table **3**); clofazimine and cycloserine were next in efficacy. Except for the carbapenems, the rest of the drugs had no statistically significant effects on treatment success and mortality. Capreomycin and kanamycin had an unfavorable benefit/toxicity ratio and are no longer recommended for the treatment of MDR/RR-TB.

Based on the result of this IPD analysis, the new WHO classification of the drugs used in the longer treatment for MDR/RR-TB is shown in Table **5**.

Table 2. Treatment regimens for poly-resistant tuberculosis*.

Pattern of Drug Resistance	Recommended Regimen	Minimum Duration of Regimen (Months)	Comments
INH-EMB	RIF+PZA+FQ	6-9	In patients with extensive disease the longer duration of treatment is recommended
INH-PZA	RIF+EMB+FQ	6-9	In patients with extensive disease the longer duration of treatment is recommended
INH-SM	RIF+EMB+PZA (±FQ)	6-9	Adding a FQ in patients with extensive disease
INH-EMB+PZA	RIF+FQ+1 SLD (LNZ or BDQ)	9-12	If LNZ or BDQ are not available a SLI could be used during the first two months

INH: isoniazid, EMB: ethambutol, PZA: pyrazinamide, SM: streptomycin, RIF: rifampin, FQ: fluoroquinolone, LNZ: linezolid, BDQ: bedaquiline, SLI: second line injectables
*modified from reference [5].

Table 3. Results from treatment correlates on outcomes in pulmonary multidrug-resistant tuberculosis: an individual patient data meta-analysis*.

Drug	Failure/Relapse *vs.* Success aOR (IC95%)	Death *vs.* Success aOR (IC95%)
[A] Levo o Moxifloxacin	0.3 (0.1-0.5)	0.2 (0.1-0.3)
[A] Bedaquiline	0.3 (0.2-0.4)	0.2 (0.2-0.3)
[A] Linezolid	0.3 (0.2-0.5)	0.3 (0.2-0.3)
[B] Clofazimine	0.3 (0.2-0.5)	0.4 (0.3-0.6)
[B] Cycloserine/Terizidone	0.6 (0.4-0.9)	0.6 (0.5-0.8)
[C] Ethambutol	0.4 (0.1-1.0)	0.5 (0.1-1.7)
[C] Delamanid	1.1 (0.4-2.8)	1.2 (0.5-3.0)
[C] Pyrazinamide	2.7 (0.7-10.9)	1.2 (0.1-15.7)
[C] Imipenem/meropenem	0.4 (0.2-0.7)	0.2 (0.1-0.5)
[C] Amikacin	0.3 (0.1-0.8)	0.7 (0.4-1.2)
[C] Streptomycin	0.5 (0.1-2.1)	0.1 (0.0-0.4)
[C] Ethionamide/Prothionamide	1.6 (0.5-5.5)	2.0 (0.8-5.3)
[C] PAS	3.1 (1.1-8.9)	1.0 (0.6-1.6)

*Modified from reference [7].

The WHO considers that under programmatic conditions, only these medicines have a role in MDR-TB treatment regimens. The use of other drugs to replace these medications could deprive a patient of a more effective treatment. Patients with very limited treatment options due to extensive resistance or lack of response to treatment may need to use medicines not included in the table. In these cases, it is recommended that the patient provides written informed consent, and health care providers strictly adhere to protocols on the management of adverse drug reactions, and data is collected to improve or develop a database on the safety and effectiveness of the medicines used.

Table 4. Serious adverse effects in the IPD meta-analysis of longer MDR-TB regimens*.

Drug	Median Risk (%) of SAE	95% Credible Interval
Bedaquiline	2.4	[0.7, 7.6]
Moxifloxacin	2.9	[1.4, 5.6]
Amoxicillin-clavulanic acid	3.0	[1.5, 5.8]
Clofazimine	3.6	[1.3, 8.6]
Ethambutol	4.0	[2.4, 6.8]
Levofloxacin	4.1	[1.9, 8.8]
Streptomycin	4.5	[2.3, 8.8]
Cycloserine/terizidone	7.8	[5.8, 10.9]
Pyrazinamide	8.8	[5.6, 13.2]
Ethionamide/prothionamide	9.5	[6.5, 14.5]
Amikacin	10.3	[6.6, 17.0]
p-aminosalicylic acid	14.3	[10.1, 20.7]
Linezolid	17.2	[10.1, 27.0]

*Modified from reference [7].

OPTIONS IN MDR-TB REGIMENS

The WHO, in its 2019 rapid communication [8], has recommended three options for the treatment of RR/MDR/XDR TB. Two are recommendations for programmatic management (the short and longer regimens) and one for operational research (the BPaL regimen):

1. For MDR/RR-TB patients without previous exposure to second-line treatment (including bedaquiline), without fluoroquinolone resistance and no extensive TB disease or severe extrapulmonary TB, the preferred treatment option is a

shorter, all-oral, bedaquiline-containing regimen (4-6 Bdq-Lfx/Mfx-Cfz-Z-E-Hh-Eto/5 Lfx/Mfx-Cfz-Z-E). Extensive (or advanced) TB disease is defined as the presence of cavitary disease, bilateral lesions, or extensive lung damage on chest radiography or multi organ-system involvement. In children under 15 years, advanced disease is usually defined by the presence of cavities or bilateral disease on chest radiography. Severe extrapulmonary TB is defined as the presence of miliary TB or TB meningitis. In children under 15 years, extrapulmonary forms of disease other than lymphadenopathy (peripheral nodes or isolated mediastinal mass without compression) are considered as severe.

2. MDR/RR-TB patients with extensive TB disease, severe forms of extrapulmonary TB, those with resistance to fluoroquinolones or who have been exposed to treatment with second-line drugs will benefit from an individualized longer regimen designed using the groups A, B, and C of drugs recommended in 2019 WHO consolidated guidelines for the treatment of drug-resistant TB.

3. The BPaL regimen (6-9 Bdq-Lzd-Pa) may be used under operational research conditions in patients with XDR-TB who have not had previous exposure to bedaquiline and linezolid (defined as less than two weeks). This regimen may not be considered for programmatic use worldwide until additional evidence on efficacy and safety has been generated. Nonetheless, in individual patients with no other options, the BPaL regimen may be used under prevailing ethical standards.

Decisions on appropriate regimens should be made based on a) results of DST, b) patient treatment history, c) severity of disease d) patient preference, and e) physician's clinical judgment.

THE SHORTER, ALL ORAL, BEDAQUILINE-CONTAINING MDR-TB REGIMEN

Up until 2016, MDR-TB treatment consisted of a standardized or individualized regimen composition with at least five medicines with an intensive phase lasting about eight months and a total length of 20 or more months. Attempts to reduce the length of treatment have been ongoing for the past 30 years. In 2016, WHO reviewed the evidence for shorter MDR-TB regimen effectiveness and safety. The evidence consisted of observational study data from 1,205 patients treated with shorter MDR-TB regimens in 10 countries in Africa and Asia. In 2017, the results of a randomized, open-label phase III, the STREAM Trial Stage 1, became available, and it was reviewed [9, 10]. As a result, in 2016, the WHO recommended a short-course (9-11 months) treatment that included a fluoroquinolone, clofazimine, ethambutol, and pyrazinamide administered over a 40-week period, supplemented by a second-line injectable, isoniazid (high dose), and prothionamide in the first 16 weeks [11]. However, as mentioned, a 2019 meta-analysis showed that the fluoroquinolones, bedaquiline, and linezolid were the three most effective drugs, while the second injectables kanamycin and capreomycin were associated with worst results and high rate of toxicity. Also, amikacin was associated with marginal efficacy and high rates of irreversible toxicity. The aim was to eliminate the injectable from the regimen due to its low efficacy and high toxicity. In 2019, based on the programmatic data of a short all-oral regimen containing bedaquiline implemented in South Africa, the WHO revised its recommendations on the use of a standardized shorter regimen. The data included a total of 10,152 records of patients with RR-/MDR-TB. The analysis compared the effectiveness of a shorter all oral bedaquilline-containing regimen to the short standardized regimen that included an injectable. Based on the analysis, WHO stated a conditional recommendation included in its new 2020 guidelines for the shorter all-oral bedaquiline-containing regimen as a treatment option to offer to MDR/RR-TB patients who satisfy the eligibility criteria:

Table 5. WHO grouping of medicines recommended for use in longer MDR-TB regimens*.

Group	Drugs	Acronym
Group A: Include all three medications unless contraindicated	Levofloxacin or Moxifloxacin Bedaquiline Linezolid	Lfx Mfx Bdq Lzd
Group B: Include one (or both)	Clofazimine Cycloserine or Terizidone	Cfz Cs Trd
Group C: Add one (s) when you cannot complete a scheme with the drugs in groups A and B	Imipenem-cilastatine Meropenem Delamanid Ethambutol Ethionamide or Prothionamide Amikacin (o Streptomycin) Pyrazinamide p-aminosalicylic acid	Ipm-Cln Mpm Dlm E Eto Pto Am (S) Z PAS

*Modified from reference [2].

A shorter, all-oral, bedaquiline-containing regimen of 9-12 months duration is recommended in eligible patients with confirmed MDR/RR-TB who have not been exposed to treatment with second-line TB medicines used in this regimen for more than one month and in whom resistance to fluoroquinolones has been excluded (Conditional recommendation, very low certainty in the evidence) [12].

It is expected that the implementation of the short-course, all-oral bedaquiline-containing MDR-TB regimen improves the programmatic management of drug-resistant TB. The regimen contains bedaquiline, levofloxacin or moxifloxacin, ethionamide or prothionamide, ethambutol, isoniazid (high-dose), pyrazinamide, and clofazimine for 4 months (with the possibility to extend to 6 months if the patient remains sputum smear-positive at the end of four months), followed by 5 months of treatment with fluoroquinolone, clofazimine, ethambutol, and pyrazinamide. Bedaquiline is used for six months minimum. All medicines are taken once a day, all days of the week. The regimen can be summarized as:

4-6 BDQ-LFX/MFX-CFZ-Z-E-H^{H}-ETO/5 LFX/MFX-CFZ-Z-E

Since the shorter all-oral bedaquiline-containing regimen was implemented as a standardized package in South Africa, it is not advisable to change the composition or shorten the duration of either phase or to prolong them in case of lack of response. The only allowed modifications are:

- If the sputum smear or cultures are still positive by the fourth month, the initial phase is prolonged until the sputum smear or culture converts; however, the initial phase is not prolonged for more than six months in total. The duration of the second phase remains fixed at five months.

- Prothionamide can be used instead of ethionamide.

- Moxifloxacin can be used instead of levofloxacin.

Any further modifications to the regimen should be done under operational research conditions.

COMPOSITION OF LONGER MDR-TB REGIMENS

WHO in its consolidated 2019 guidelines [2] recommends for the longer regimens:

1. In MDR/RR-TB patients on longer regimens, all three Group A agents and at least one Group B agent should be included to ensure that treatment starts with at least four TB agents likely to be active and that at least three agents are included for the rest of therapy after bedaquiline is stopped.

2. If only one or two Group A agents are used, both Group B agents are to be included.

3. If the regimen cannot be composed with agents from Groups A and B alone, Group C agents are added to complete it.

4. Kanamycin and capreomycin are not to be included in the treatment of MDR/RR-TB patients on longer regimens.

5. Levofloxacin or moxifloxacin should be included in the treatment of MDR/RR-TB patients on longer regimens.

6. Bedaquiline should be included in longer MDR-TB regimens for patients aged 18 years or more. Bedaquiline may also be included in longer MDR-TB regimens for patients aged 6–17 years.

7. Linezolid should be included in the treatment of MDR/RR-TB patients on longer regimens.

8. Clofazimine and cycloserine or terizidone may be included in the treatment of MDR/RR-TB patients on longer regimens.

9. Ethambutol may be included in the treatment of MDR/RR-TB patients on longer regimens.

10. Delamanid may be included in the treatment of MDR/RR-TB patients aged three years or more on longer regimens [13].

11. Pyrazinamide may be included in the treatment of MDR/RR-TB patients on longer regimens. Z is only counted as an effective agent when DST results confirm susceptibility.

12. Imipenem–cilastatin or meropenem may be included in the treatment of MDR/RR-TB patients.

13. Amikacin may be included in the treatment of MDR/RR-TB patients aged 18 years or more on longer regimens when susceptibility has been demonstrated and adequate measures to monitor for adverse reactions can be ensured. If amikacin is not available, streptomycin may replace amikacin under the same conditions.

14. Ethionamide or prothionamide may be included in the treatment of MDR/RR-

TB patients on longer regimens only if bedaquiline, linezolid, clofazimine or delamanid are not used or if better options to compose a regimen are not possible.

15. p-aminosalicylic acid may be included in the treatment of MDR/RR-TB patients on longer regimens only if bedaquiline, linezolid, clofazimine or delamanid are not used or if better options to compose a regimen are not possible.

16. Clavulanic acid should not be included in the treatment of MDR/RR-TB patients on longer regimens unless it is used with a β-lactamic.

Table 6. Daily dosage of drugs in the all oral short course treatment with bedaquiline BDQ (100 mg tablets) is given 4 tablets daily for two weeks and subsequently 2 tablets 3 times a week for 22 weeks*.

Drug	Tablet	30-35 kg	36-45 kg	46-55 kg	56-70 kg	>70 kg
Mfx	400 mg	1	1	1	1	1
Lfx	250 mg	3	3	4	4	4
	500 mg	1.5	1.5	2	2	2
	750 mg	1	1	1.5	1.5	1,5
Cfz	50 mg	2	2	2	2	2
	100 mg	1	1	1	1	1
Emb	400 mg	2	2	3	3	3
PZA	400 mg	3	4	4	4	5
	500 mg	2	3	3	3	4
INH	100 mg	2	3	3	3	3
	300 mg	2/3	1	1	1	1
ETO/PTO	250 mg	2	2	3	3	4

*modified from reference [12].

Subgroup Considerations

MDR/RR-TB in People Living with HIV

The treatment regimen for MDR/RR-TB is the same for people living with HIV. Attention should be paid to potential interactions between antituberculosis drugs and antiretrovirals (see Chapter 9; Tuberculosis in persons living with HIV). Thioacetazone (no longer on the WHO list of essential medications for tuberculosis) should be avoided in patients with HIV because of the risk of Stevens-Johnson syndrome and toxic epidermal necrolysis [7].

MDR/RR-TB Alone or with Additional Resistance

Any regimen for drug-resistant TB is more likely to be effective if its composition is based on information from reliable drug susceptibility testing. Ideally, all patients with MDR/RR-TB should be tested for resistance to fluoroquinolones as a minimum before the start of the treatment. If the patient is going to be treated with the short-course regimen (see Short-Course Treatment for MDR/RR-TB in the following pages), rapid testing for second-line injectable should also be performed.

Rifampin-Resistant TB

Patients with RR-TB but without isoniazid resistance need to be treated with a recommended MDR-TB regimen to which isoniazid is added.

Children

The WHO recommendations on longer MDR-TB regimens also apply to children. As mentioned, bedaquiline can be used in children six years of age and older, and delamanid in children three years of age and older. The avoidance of an injectable is especially desirable in children since hearing loss can have a permanent effect on the acquisition of language and school performance. If an injectable is needed due to the non-availability or toxicity of drugs from groups A and B, the availability of audiometry testing is indispensable [14].

Extrapulmonary TB and TB Meningitis

The WHO longer MDR-TB treatment regimen also applies to patients with extrapulmonary TB. The fluoroquinolones, ethionamide/prothionamide, cycloserine/terizidone, linezolid, high dose isoniazid, pyrazinamide, and imipenem-cilastatin penetrate well into the central nervous system. Amikacin and streptomycin penetrate well into the CNS but only in the presence of meningeal inflammation. Meropenem is preferred in children with TB meningitis since imipenem is associated with seizures in pediatric patients.

In MDR/RR-TB patients on longer regimens, a total treatment duration of 18–20 months is suggested for most patients; the length may be modified according to the patient's response to therapy. In MDR/RR-TB patients on longer regimens, a treatment duration of 15–17 months after culture conversion is suggested for most patients. In MDR/RR-TB patients on longer regimens that contain an injectable, an intensive phase of 6–7 months is suggested for most patients; the duration may be modified according to the patient's response to therapy.

The performance of sputum culture in addition to sputum smear microscopy is recommended for monitor treatment response. It is desirable for sputum culture to be repeated at monthly intervals.

Electrocardiography should be included in the monitoring protocol since regimens will have two or three agents that are expected to prolong the QT (bedaquiline, delamanid, fluoroquinolones, and clofazimine).

BPAL REGIMEN FOR TREATMENT OF MDR/RR-TB WITH ADDITIONAL FLUOROQUINOLONE RESISTANCE

Patients with extensive resistance patterns have very limited treatment options and a cure rate under 40%.

Recently, an open-label, one-arm study was carried out in South Africa with an all-oral regimen that included three drugs: bedaquiline, pretomanid, and linezolid, drugs that have bactericidal and sterilizing activity against *M. tuberculosis*. The regimen can be summarized as 6-9 BDQ-Pa-Lzd.

The study was designed to evaluate the safety and efficacy of this drug combination for 26 weeks in patients with extensively drug-resistant tuberculosis (XDR-TB) and patients with multidrug-resistant tuberculosis with poor response to treatment or for which a second-line regimen had been discontinued because of side effects. The primary endpoint was the rate of an unfavorable outcome, defined as treatment failure or relapse during follow-up, which continued until six months after the end of the treatment.

One hundred and nine patients were enrolled in the study. At the end of the treatment, 11 patients (10%) had an unfavorable outcome, and 98 patients (90%; 95% confidence interval, 83 to 95) had a favorable outcome. The 11 unfavorable outcomes included seven deaths, one withdrawal of consent during the treatment, two relapses during follow-up, and one loss to follow-up.

Linezolid toxic effects of peripheral neuropathy were reported in 81% of patients and myelosuppression in 48%, often leading to dose reductions or interruptions in the treatment with linezolid [15]. There were signals of reproductive toxicity with the potential effects on human male fertility that have been observed in the preclinical data from animal studies [12].

After considering the evidence, especially the small sample size and the high rate of serious adverse effects, the WHO has recommended that the BPaL regimen should be used under operational research conditions, and not for programmatic implementation:

A treatment regimen lasting 6-9 months composed of bedaquiline, pretomanid and linezolid (BPaL) may be used under operational research conditions in MDR-TB patients with TB resistant to fluoroquinolones and who have had no previous exposure to bedaquiline and linezolid for more than two weeks. (conditional recommendation, very low certainty in the estimates of effect).

A patient could be eligible for treatment with the BPaL regimen if:

1. Is diagnosed with confirmed resistance to rifampicin and fluoroquinolones with/without resistance to injectable agents.

2. Is ≥14 years of age.

3. Weighs ≥35kg or more.

4. Gives informed consent to be enrolled in the operational research project.

5. Non-pregnant or non-breastfeeding females that are willing to use effective contraception.

6. With no known allergies to the drugs included in the regimen.

7. The patient has not been exposed to a strain resistant to the drugs included in the regimen.

8. The patient has not received the drugs included in the regimen for ≥2 weeks.

9. The patient has no extrapulmonary TB (including meningitis, other central nervous system TB, or TB osteomyelitis).

People Living with HIV Infection (PLHIV)

People living with HIV infection represented half of those enrolled in the Nix-TB study. PLHIV were eligible to enroll in the Nix-TB study if they had a CD4 count of >50 cells/μL and if they were using antiretroviral medications. It is essential to note drug-drug interactions when administering TB and HIV medications in combination, including the documented interactions between bedaquiline with efavirenz and ritonavir.

Patients with Very Limited Treatment Options

In patients with extensive drug resistance, it might be difficult to construct a regimen based on existing recommendations. In such situations, the BPaL regimen may be considered as a last resort under prevailing ethical standards.

REFERENCES

[1]   Laniado-Laborín R. El ABC de la tuberculosis resistente a los fármacos: Manual práctico de diagnóstico y tratamiento Capítulo 4: Tratamiento de la tuberculosis resistente a fármacos. Editorial Académica Española 2012; pp. 19-23. ISBN-103848459884.

[2]   WHO. consolidated guidelines on tuberculosis. Module 4: treatment - drug-resistant tuberculosis treatment. Geneva: World Health Organization 2020. Licence: CC BY-NC-SA 3.0 IGO.

[3]   Zaragoza B, Laniado-Laborín R. Diagnosing drug-resistant tuberculosis with the xpert®MTB/RIF. The risk for rifampin susceptible cases. J Tuberc Res 2017; 5: 155-60.
        [http://dx.doi.org/10.4236/jtr.2017.53017]

[4]   Menzies D, Benedetti A, Paydar A, *et al.* Standardized treatment of active tuberculosis in patients with previous treatment and/or with mono-resistance to isoniazid: a systematic review and meta-analysis. PLoS Med 2009; 6(9): e1000150.
        [http://dx.doi.org/10.1371/journal.pmed.1000150] [PMID: 20101802]

[5]   Curry international tuberculosis center and california department of public health. Drug-Resistant Tuberculosis: A Survival Guide for Clinicians. 3rd ed. 2016; pp. 67-9.

[6]   WHO. Global tuberculosis report. Geneva: World Health Organization; 2018 (WHO/CDS/TB/201820 2018. http://apps.who.int/iris/bitstream/handle/10665/274453/9789241 565646-eng.pdf

[7]   Ahmad N, Ahuja SD, Akkerman OW, *et al.* Collaborative Group for the Meta-Analysis of Individual Patient Data in MDR-TB treatment–2017. Treatment correlates of successful outcomes in pulmonary multidrug-resistant tuberculosis: an individual patient data meta-analysis. Lancet 2018; 392(10150): 821-34.
        [http://dx.doi.org/10.1016/S0140-6736(18)31644-1] [PMID: 30215381]

[8]   Rapid Communication on forthcoming changes to the programmatic management of tuberculosis preventive treatment. Geneva: World Health Organization 2020. (WHO/UCN/TB/2020.4). Licence: CC BY-NC-SA 3.0 IGO.

[9]   Nunn A, Rusen ID, Van Deun A, *et al.* Evaluation of a standardized treatment regimen of anti-tuberculosis drugs for patients with multi-drug-resistant tuberculosis (STREAM): study protocol for a randomized controlled trial. Trials 2014 Sep; 9;15: 353.
        [http://dx.doi.org/10.1186/1745-6215-15-353] [PMID: 25199531]

[10]   Nunn AJ, Phillips PPJ, Meredith SK, *et al.* STREAM Study Collaborators. A trial of a shorter regimen for rifampin-resistant tuberculosis. N Engl J Med 2019; 380(13): 1201-13.
        [http://dx.doi.org/10.1056/NEJMoa1811867] [PMID: 30865791]

[11]   WHO. Treatment guidelines for drug-resistant tuberculosis – 2016 update. World Health Organization 2016. WHO/HTM/TB/2016.04.

[12]   World Health Organization. WHO consolidated guidelines on tuberculosis Module 4: Drug Resistant Tuberculosis Treatment. Geneva: World Health Organization 2020.

[13]   World Health Organization. The use of delamanid in the treatment of multidrug-resistant tuberculosis in children and adolescents: interim policy guidance 2016. ISBN 978 92 4 154989 9

[14]   Harausz EP, Garcia-Prats AJ, Law S, *et al.* Collaborative Group for Meta-Analysis of Paediatric

Individual Patient Data in MDR-TB. Treatment and outcomes in children with multidrug-resistant tuberculosis: A systematic review and individual patient data meta-analysis. PLoS Med 2018; 15(7): e1002591.
[http://dx.doi.org/10.1371/journal.pmed.1002591] [PMID: 29995958]

[15]   Conradie F, Diacon AH, Ngubane N, *et al.* Nix-TB Trial Team. Treatment of highly drug-resistant pulmonary tuberculosis. N Engl J Med 2020; 382(10): 893-902.
[http://dx.doi.org/10.1056/NEJMoa1901814] [PMID: 32130813]

CHAPTER 12

Diagnosis and Treatment of Latent Tuberculosis Infection

Abstract: One-third of the world's population is infected with *M. tuberculosis*. It is from this vast pool of infected people where the new cases of active disease originate. Most of these cases of latent infection are found in low-income countries where national tuberculosis programs concentrate practically all their efforts on the diagnosis and treatment of tuberculosis disease, neglecting the diagnosis and treatment of latent tuberculosis in contacts of an active case. Each case of pulmonary tuberculosis infects an average of 20 contacts, and of these, 10% of immunocompetent subjects will develop the active disease if the latent infection is not detected and treated, which means that each case of active TB will generate two new cases of TB; this explains, at least in part, the difficulty that high burden countries have in controlling the epidemic. These figures are even higher for subjects with some state of immunosuppression (for example, people living with HIV, patients receiving immunosuppressive treatment, malnourished, *etc.*).

For the diagnosis of latent TB, we currently have *in vitro* tests to determine the release of interferon-γ (IGRA´s), with higher specificity than the traditional tuberculin test, an essential point in subjects vaccinated with BCG.

Also, now there is a regimen (isoniazid and rifapentine) that requires only 12 doses of medication instead of 180-270 doses of isoniazid, which facilitates adherence to the regimen, with the same effectiveness and less toxicity.

The WHO has recommended the treatment of infected cases of MDR-TB (specifically children and people living with HIV) with a fluoroquinolone.

Keywords: HIV, IGRA, Infection, Isoniazid, Latent, Rifapentine, Treatment, Tuberculin, Tuberculosis.

INTRODUCTION

The control of an epidemic secondary to an infectious disease requires the following steps:

1. Active search for cases.

2. When possible, treatment of cases.

3. Interruption of the transmission chain.

4. Improvement of the immune response of susceptible subjects.

However, if the eradication of the disease is desired, it is necessary to eliminate the reservoir of the infection [1].

Latent tuberculosis infection (LTBI) is defined as the persistent immune response to the stimulation of *Mycobacterium tuberculosis* (MTB) antigens without the presence of clinical manifestations of active tuberculosis disease (TB) in a person who has acquired the infection from an active case of TB. Although this condition is not infectious, subjects with LTBI are at risk of developing active TB and are able to transmit the infection to their contacts. The lifelong risk of reactivation of TB in an immunocompetent individual with LTBI is estimated at 5-15%, especially during the 5 years after acquiring the infection. However, the risk of activation is much higher in immunocompromised individuals, as is the case of people living with HIV/AIDS [2].

The most recent estimates of LTBI indicate that approximately 1.7 billion people are infected worldwide, 10% of whom are infected with an isoniazid-resistant strain. Preventing people infected with MTB from progressing to developing the active disease is essential to reduce the rates of morbidity and mortality occuring due to TB [3]. If we do not diagnose and treat LTBI efficiently, the ambitious goal of the World Health Organization (WHO) End of Tuberculosis strategy to reduce the incidence of TB by 90% (less than 10 cases per 100,000 h), by the year 2035, will not be reached [4].

Although it is still necessary to aggressively find and treat all TB cases effectively to stop the chain of transmission in the community, this strategy will not be enough since it does not address the enormous reservoir of infected individuals that eventually (about 10%) will reactivate and become infectious [5]. It is estimated that every infectious TB case will infect approximately 20 contacts, of which 2 (10%) will progress to active disease, with an exponential increase in infected and diseased individuals with the passage of time. The WHO now recognizes that to reach the End TB goals, it will require a worldwide effort to address LTBI [6].

The most recent guidelines of the WHO for the programmatic management of LTBI are mainly directed to countries with TB incidence lower than 100 cases per 100,000 population. However, it is evident that any country, regardless of its TB rate, can benefit from the management systematized of the LTBI. The most recent WHO guide focuses on middle and high-income countries because according to this document, these countries can potentially benefit more from the programmatic management of LTBI, taking into account their current epidemiological situation, their availability of resources and the fact that most cases in these countries are a result of te reactivation of the LTBI and not from the recent transmission from an active case [2].

HIGH-RISK GROUPS FOR LTBI DIAGNOSIS AND TREATMENT

Not all individuals with LTBI progress to active disease. Given that the treatment of LTBI represents costs and potential risks of adverse reactions to the medication used, it is recommended that the treatment of LTBI be selectively focused on those groups with greater risk of progression to active disease, which will obtain the maximum benefit when receiving treatment for LTBI. Two particularly vulnerable groups are children under 5 years of age and those with immunological compromise [6].

Populations at risk for whom diagnosis and treatment of LTBI are recommended by the WHO [6]:

1. **Adults and adolescents living with HIV/AIDS:** TB is the leading cause of death in patients with HIV, accounting for a third of all deaths in this population group. Randomized studies have shown that preventive therapy in this group reduces the risk of developing active TB in 33% and 64% in subjects with HIV and positive tuberculin test. The treatment of LTBI combined with antiretroviral treatment (ART) has an additive effect in reducing the incidence and mortality, an effect that lasts for at least 5 years.

2. **Infants and children living with HIV/AIDS:** Children under one year of age living with HIV who are in contact with a case of active TB and who do not present clinical data of active disease should receive preventive treatment. Children older than one year of age living with HIV in a region with a high prevalence of TB and who are not at risk of infection based on clinical data and absence of contact with a TB case should be offered treatment with isoniazid for six months as part of a comprehensive package of prevention in HIV.

3. **Home contacts of an active TB case:** All household contacts, regardless of their age or LTBI status, are at higher risk of progression to active TB than the

general population. Children under five years of age, household contacts of patients with bacteriologically confirmed TB, and who do not have active TB (based on an adequate clinical evaluation) should receive preventive treatment; this group has the highest risk of disseminated TB. In countries with a low TB burden, all household contacts of people with bacteriologically confirmed TB should be studied and receive preventive treatment if they are infected. In countries with high incidence, home contacts of a bacteriologically confirmed case could receive preventive therapy according to the WHO recommendations.

4. **Other at-risk groups:** Patients with immunosuppression, including those who will initiate treatment with anti-TNF biologics, patients on hemodialysis, patients awaiting hematological transplantation, and patients with silicosis should be systematically studied and treated for LTBI. Although this is a WHO recommendation, the quality of the evidence is very low. In countries with low incidence (<100 cases per 100,000 h.), prisoners, health workers, migrants from regions with high incidence, homeless people, and users of illicit drugs can be considered for diagnosis and treatment of LTBI. The WHO recommendation for this last group is conditional due to the low quality of the evidence.

TESTING FOR LTBI

We do not have a gold standard for the diagnosis of LTBI, and it is diagnosed indirectly by detecting the immune response of the subject to the antigens of MTB; in fact, we do not know if at, the time of the test, the infected subject still has viable mycobacteria in his/her tissues. Both the tuberculin skin test (TST) and interferon-gamma release assays (IGRAs) require an active immune response to identify those who are infected with *M. tuberculosis* and are not useful in predicting the progression of infection to disease.

TUBERCULIN SKIN TEST

The tuberculin test is based on the fact that infection with *M. tuberculosis* produces a late hypersensitivity response to some of the antigenic components of mycobacteria, which are present in extracts of filtrates of MTB cultures.

The reaction to the intradermal application of tuberculin is the classic example of delayed cellular hypersensitivity. T cells that have been previously sensitized by infection with MTB are recruited to the site of cutaneous injection where they release cytokines. These induce an induration process through local vasodilation, edema, fibrin deposition, recruitment of other inflammatory cells with occasional vesiculation, and necrosis [7]. The reaction is characterized by its slow course, reaching its maximum induration after 24 hours of tuberculin application.

Purified protein derivative tuberculin (PPD) is obtained from a mycobacterial culture filtrate by protein precipitation; it also contains some polysaccharides and small amounts of lipids. Most of the PPD proteins are small and, therefore, do not sensitize the infected subject with its cutaneous application.

PPD, when diluted, is adsorbed by glass and plastic, therefore, a detergent (Tween 80) is added to reduce this effect. Therefore, the tuberculin test should be carried out shortly after loading the reagent into the syringe. PPD must be kept refrigerated and avoid exposure to sunlight.

The tuberculin test is carried out by injecting 0.1 mL of PPD 5 TU intradermally in the anterior surface of the forearm using a tuberculin syringe (1 mL capacity and 27-gauge needle) with the bevel of the needle up; the correct application will produce a 6-10 mm diameter papule. The response is read between 48 and 72 hours after the application. The reaction is measured in millimeters of induration (palpable papule). Erythema is not considered. The diameter of the induration area is measured in millimeters along the transverse axis of the forearm.

The interpretation of the results of the TST depends on the degree of induration in millimeters and the risk of the subject progressing to active disease in case of being infected [6].

An induration of 5 millimeters or more is considered positive in people living with HIV/AIDS, in recent contacts of an active case, in people with fibrotic changes compatible with TB on chest radiography, in patients with organ transplants, and, in general, in people with immunosuppression (TNF alpha antagonists, immunosuppressant therapy, *etc.*).

An induration of 10 or more millimeters is considered positive in recent migrants (<5 years) from regions with high prevalence, users of illicit drugs, residents and employees of hospices or asylums, and people with clinical conditions that put them at risk [8].

The sensitivity of the tuberculin test to detect infection is approximately 70-75% (determined in patients with bacteriologically confirmed tuberculosis). False negatives are frequent in immunocompromised individuals. False positives may occur in individuals who are infected with non-tuberculous mycobacteria or who have been vaccinated with BCG. The impact of BCG vaccination on the specificity of TST depends on several factors, including the strain of vaccine used, the age at which the vaccine is given, and the number of doses administered. When BCG is given at birth, as is the case in most parts of the world, it has a variable and limited impact on TST specificity in older children and adults [8].

Interferon-gamma (IFN-γ) release assays are known by the acronym IGRAs. IGRAs are in-vitro assays and constitute an alternative to TST. They are based on the detection of the response of T cells to antigens specific to *M. tuberculosis*. To date, there are two commercial IGRAs available: the QuantiFERON-TB (QFTB) and the T-SPOT TB.

The QFTB uses a peptide combination that simulates *M. tuberculosis* proteins to stimulate cells in whole blood to release IFN-γ. The response to specific *M. tuberculosis* proteins, including the early secretory antigenic target-6 (ESAT-6) and culture filtrate protein 10 (CFP-10) with the liberation of IFN-γ is measured by enzyme-linked immunosorbent assay (ELISA). ESAT-6 and CFP-10 are present in *M. tuberculosis* and stimulate a measurable release of IFN-γ in infected individuals; they are absent in BCG vaccine strains and in most non-tuberculous mycobacteria, a feature that confers the test higher specificity. These proteins are present in *M. kansasii*, *M. szulgai*, and *M. marinum* and could cause false-positive IGRA results [9].

The most recent version of the QFTB and QuantiFERON-TB Gold Plus, has replaced the previous version, the QuantiFERON GOLD in the tube. It contains specific CD8 antigens in a new tube explicitly designed to stimulate CD8+ and CD4+ T cells. This extra tube complements the tubes that contain ESAT-6 and CFP-10 that determine the response of CD4+ cells and T-helper cells [10]. (Kamada, 2017). The sensitivity of this new version is 90-94%, and its specificity is 99% (Table **1**).

The test is reported as positive, negative, or indeterminate (indeterminate tests must be repeated).

Table 1. Interpretation of a QuantiFERON TB Gold plus test.

Nil (IU/mL)	TB1-Nil (IU/mL)	TB2-Nil (IU/mL)	Mitogen-Nil (IU/mL)	QFT-Plus results
≤ 8.0	≥ 0.35 and ≥0.25 of Nil	Any	Any	Positive
	Any	≥ 0.35 and ≥0.25 of Nil		
	<0.35 or ≥ 0.35 and <0.25 of Nil	<0.35 or ≥0.25 and <25% of Nil	≥ 0.50	Negative
	<0.35 or ≥ 0.35 and <0.25 of Nil	<0.35 or ≥ 0.35 and <0.25 of Nil	<0.50	Indeterminate
>8.0	Any			

The T-SPOT test is designed to detect effector T cells that respond to *M. tuberculosis*-specific antigens (ESAT-6 and CFP-10); the points observed in the activated T cells are counted in the assay. The test uses the peripheral mononuclear cells of the patient's blood that are incubated with the antigens to facilitate the stimulation of activated T cells. Each point represents the fingerprint of response to stimulation with specific antigens and provides an estimate of the abundance of sensitized effector T cells in peripheral blood. The results of the T-SPOT are interpreted by subtracting the number of points in the cells of the null control well from those present in the wells with antigen. The test is considered positive if the count of the points in at least one of the wells with antigen minus the points on the null well is ≥6 [9].

The WHO recommendations 2020 guideline are as follow (Table **2**) [6]:

1. Either a tuberculin skin test (TST) or interferon-gamma release assay (IGRA) can be used to test for LTBI. This is considered a strong recommendation despite very low-quality evidence.

2. People living with HIV who have a positive test for LTBI benefit more from preventive treatment than those who have a negative LTBI test; LTBI testing can be used, where feasible, to identify such individuals. This a strong recommendation based on high-quality evidence.

3. LTBI testing by TST or IGRA is not a requirement for initiating preventive treatment in people living with HIV or child household contacts aged <5 years. (Strong recommendation, moderate-quality evidence).

Also, the WHO in its guideline states that the availability and affordability of the tests will determine which will be chosen by clinicians and program managers. *Neither TST nor IGRA can be used to diagnose active TB disease nor for diagnostic workup of adults suspected of having active TB*.

Table 2. Recommended dosages of drugs for the treatment of LTBI*.

Drug Regimen	Dose/kg/Body Weight	Maximum Dose
Isoniazid (daily for 6-9 months)	Adults 5 mg/kg Children 10 mg/kg	300 mg
Rifampin (daily for 3-4 months)	Adults 10 mg/kg Children 15 mg/kg	600 mg
Isoniazid + Rifampin (daily for 3-4 months	Isoniazid: Adults 5 mg Children 10 mg Rifampin Adults 10 mg Children 15 mg	Isoniazid 300 mg Rifampin 600 mg

(Table 2) cont.....

Drug Regimen	Dose/kg/Body Weight	Maximum Dose
Weekly rifapentine plus isoniazid for 3 months (12 doses)	Individuals ≥ 12 years: isoniazid: 15 mg Individuals 2–11 years: isoniazid: 25 mg Rifapentine: 10.0–14.0 kg = 300 mg 14.1–25.0 kg = 450 mg 25.1–32.0 kg = 600 mg 32.1–50.0 kg = 750 mg > 50 kg = 900 mg	Isoniazid 900 mg Rifapentine 900 mg

*Modified from reference [6].

TREATMENT OF LATENT TUBERCULOSIS INFECTIONS

The WHO published, in 2020, the following recommendations [6]:

1. The following options are recommended for the treatment of LTBI regardless of HIV status: 6 or 9 months of daily isoniazid, or a 3-month regimen of weekly rifapentine plus isoniazid, or a 3-month regimen of daily isoniazid plus rifampicin. (Strong recommendation, moderate to high certainty in the estimates of effect).

2. A 1-month regimen of daily rifapentine plus isoniazid or 4 months of daily rifampicin alone may also be offered as alternatives. (Conditional recommendation, low to moderate certainty in the estimates of effect).

3. In settings with high TB transmission, adults and adolescents living with HIV who have an unknown or a positive LTBI test and are unlikely to have active TB disease should receive at least 36 months of daily isoniazid preventive treatment (IPT). Daily IPT for 36 months should be given whether or not the person is on ART, and irrespective of the degree of immunosuppression, history of previous TB treatment, and pregnancy, in settings considered to have a high TB transmission as defined by national authorities. (Conditional recommendation, low certainty in the estimates of effect).

The original publication [11] compared three months of rifapentine and isoniazid (RP-H) once a week under direct observations *vs.* isoniazid (H) for 9 months, self-administered. The rate of active TB in the RP-H group was 0.19% *vs.* 0.43% in the H group; rates of treatment completion were 82.1% for the RP-H group *vs.* 69.0% in the H group (p<0.001). The rate of permanent discontinuation due to adverse effects was higher in the RP-H group (4.9% *vs.* 3.7%, p=0.009). Drug hepatotoxicity was more frequent in the H group (2.7% *vs.* 0.4, p<0.001). This same regimen was studied in children [12] in a multicenter study conducted in 29 sites in the USA, Canada, Brazil, China, and Spain. Participants were aged 2-17 years. RP-H 12 doses, once a week, under direct supervision was compared with H (270 daily doses, unsupervised). In the RP-H group (471 children), 88.1% completed treatment while 80.9% of the 434 children completed treatment in the H (p=0.003); adverse effects were more common in the RP-H group (0.6% *vs.* 0.2%). There were no severe hepatotoxicity cases or deaths in either of the groups. None of the RP-H group participants and 3 of the 434 in the H group developed active TB (0.74%).

The Centers for Disease Control (CDC) in the United States conducted a systematic review and meta-analyses of the RP-H regimen, which determined that RP-H is as safe and effective as other recommended LTBI regimens and achieves substantially higher treatment completion rates [13]. The CDC now recommends the RP-H regimen for treatment of LTBI in adults, in children with LTBI aged 2–17 years, and in individuals with LTBI who have HIV/AIDS and are taking antiretroviral medications with acceptable drug-drug interactions with rifapentine.

For countries with low TB incidence, the WHO recommends the following options for LTBI treatment as alternatives to 6 months of isoniazid monotherapy [6]:

1. 9 months of isoniazid.

2. A 3-month regimen of weekly rifapentine plus isoniazid.

3. 3–4 months of isoniazid plus rifampicin.

4. 3–4 months of rifampicin alone.

5. In settings with high TB incidence and transmission, adults and adolescents living with HIV who have an unknown or a positive LTBI test in whom active TB has been ruled out should receive at least 36 months of isoniazid therapy, regardless of whether they are receiving antiretroviral therapy.

This last recommendation is based on a systematic review and meta-analysis from 49 articles from the literature and three studies conducted in Bostwana, South Africa, and India. The risk of active TB was 38% lower among patients receiving 36 months of continuous isoniazid compared with the isoniazid regimen for 6 months; the benefit was even stronger (49% lower risk of active TB) for individuals with a positive tuberculin skin test. Mortality for subjects with a positive skin test was 50% lower. Two of the studies found no evidence of an increase in adverse events in the continuous isoniazid group, whereas the other found strong evidence of an increase. The analysis reported no evidence of increased drug resistance when continuous isoniazid was given [14].

A new regimen for patients with HIV and TB co-infection consists of rifapentine (at a dose of 300 mg daily for patients weighing 35-44 kg, 450 mg daily for patients weighing 35 to 45 kg, and 600 mg for patients weighing more than 45 kilograms), plus isoniazid at a dose of 300 mg daily for 1 month. This regimen was compared to a 36-week regimen of isoniazid alone at a dose of 300 mg daily and proved not to be inferior. A total of 3,000 patients were enrolled in this study and followed for a median of 3.3 years. The median CD4+ cell count was 470 cells/mL^3, and half the patients were receiving antiretroviral therapy. The primary endpoint was a diagnosis of tuberculosis or death from tuberculosis or an unknown cause during follow-up, and it was reported to be 2% in the rifapentine-isoniazid group and 2% in the isoniazid group, for an incidence rate of 0.65 per 100 person-years and 0.67 per 100 person-years, respectively. Serious adverse events occurred in 6% of the patients in the rifapentine-isoniazid group and in 7% of those in the isoniazid group (p=0.07). However, the percentage of treatment completion was significantly higher in the rifapentine-isoniazid group than in the isoniazid group (97% *vs.* 90%, p<0.001) [15].

PREVENTIVE TREATMENT IN CONTACTS OF PATIENTS WITH MULTIDRUG-RESISTANT TUBERCULOSIS

Considering the dire consequences of developing MDR-TB, finally, the policy of "watch and wait" has been replaced by recommendations by international agencies for the treatment of LTBI in MDR-TB contacts [16].

Obviously, isoniazid and rifampin must be considered ineffective in MDR cases. Fluoroquinolones, a drug group that has been used extensively for the treatment of drug-resistant TB, improving patient outcomes, has shown good efficacy in the laboratory against *M. tuberculosis* with excellent early bactericidal activity (EBA).

Originally there was concern about the safety of fluoroquinolones in children from data reported in old animal studies; however, these drugs have been used extensively and safely in children with drug-resistant tuberculosis.

The likelihood that a contact might be infected with the same strain harbored by the index case is determined by several factors, including the degree of infectiousness of the index case and the intensity and duration of exposure. This is likely to be higher in small children whose social circle is very limited beyond that of the index case.

Another critical concern regarding the use of fluoroquinolones for LTBI contacts is the possibility of resistance propagation. If the active disease is carefully excluded, the low number of mycobacteria present in LTBI makes the development of resistance highly unlikely. Spontaneous mutations associated with isoniazid resistance occur once every 10^{5-6} divisions [17], while mutations causing resistance to fluoroquinolones arise even less frequently (about every 10^{6-8} divisions) [18].

The WHO, in its 2018 LTBI treatment guidelines [6], recommends that *"in selected high-risk household contacts of patients with multidrug-resistant tuberculosis, preventive treatment may be considered based on individualized risk assessment and sound clinical justification."* This is a conditional recommendation due to the very low quality of the evidence. The recommendation includes only household contacts at high risk (children, people living with HIV/AIDS, and other immunocompromised individuals), and confirmation of infection with LTBI test is required. The WHO also recommends strict clinical observation and close monitoring for the development of active TB disease for at least 2 years, regardless of the provision or not of preventive treatment.

As the recommendation is based on very low-quality evidence, WHO suggests that the subjects must be given detailed information about the benefits and harms of the preventive treatment and asked for explicit written informed consent.

Later-generation fluoroquinolones (*e.g.* levofloxacin and moxifloxacin) are the drugs recommended for preventive treatment in MDR-TB cases unless the strain of the index case is resistant to these drugs. Levofloxacin is preferred over moxifloxacin due to its lower toxicity and cost. The duration of this regimen, due to the very limited evidence, should be based on clinical judgment and could be administered for 6, 9, or 12 months.

REFERENCES

[1]   Rangaka MX, Cavalcante SC, Marais BJ, *et al.* Controlling the seedbeds of tuberculosis: diagnosis and treatment of tuberculosis infection. Lancet 2015; 386(10010): 2344-53.
[http://dx.doi.org/10.1016/S0140-6736(15)00323-2] [PMID: 26515679]

[2]   Laniado-Laborín R. Why has the management of latent tuberculosis been relegated in high burden countries? an ounce of prevention is worth a pound of cure. J Respir Res 2018; 4: 134-6.
[http://dx.doi.org/10.17554/j.issn.2412-2424.2018.04.38]

[3]   Global tuberculosis report 2017. Geneva: World Health Organization 2017. Licence: CC BY-NCSA 3.0 IGO.

[4]   Houben RM, Dodd PJ. The global burden of latent tuberculosis infection: a re-estimation using mathematical modelling. PLoS Med 2016 Oct 25; 13(10): e1002152.
[http://dx.doi.org/10.1371/journal.pmed.1002152] [PMID: 27780211]

[5]   Badje A, Moh R, Gabillard D, *et al.* Temprano ANRS 12136 Study Group. Effect of isoniazid preventive therapy on risk of death in west African, HIV-infected adults with high CD4 cell counts: long-term follow-up of the Temprano ANRS 12136 trial. Lancet Glob Health 2017; 5(11): e1080-9. [http://dx.doi.org/10.1016/S2214-109X(17)30372-8] [PMID: 29025631]

[6]   WHO. consolidated guidelines on tuberculosis Module 1: prevention – tuberculosis preventive treatment Geneva: World Health Organization 2020. Licence: CC BY-NC-SA 3.0 IGO.

[7]   Colvin RB, Mosesson MW, Dvorak HF. Delayed-type hypersensitivity skin reactions in congenital afibrinogenemia lack fibrin deposition and induration. J Clin Invest 1979; 63(6): 1302-6. [http://dx.doi.org/10.1172/JCI109425] [PMID: 447844]

[8]   Testing for TB Infection. Factsheet, Centers for Disease Control. https://www.cdc.gov/tb/topic/test ing/tbtesttypes.htm

[9]   Moon HW, Hur M. Interferon-gamma release assays for the diagnosis of latent tuberculosis infection: an updated review. Ann Clin Lab Sci 2013; 43(2): 221-9. [PMID: 23694799]

[10]   Kamada A, Amishima M. QuantiFERON-TB® Gold Plus as a potential tuberculosis treatment monitoring tool. Eur Respir J 2017; 49(3): 1601976. [http://dx.doi.org/10.1183/13993003.01976-2016] [PMID: 28331040]

[11]   Sterling TR, Villarino ME, Borisov AS, *et al.* TB Trials Consortium PREVENT TB Study Team. Three months of rifapentine and isoniazid for latent tuberculosis infection. N Engl J Med 2011; 365(23): 2155-66. [http://dx.doi.org/10.1056/NEJMoa1104875] [PMID: 22150035]

[12]   Villarino ME, Scott NA, Weis SE, *et al.* International Maternal Pediatric and Adolescents AIDS Clinical Trials Group; Tuberculosis Trials Consortium. Treatment for preventing tuberculosis in children and adolescents: a randomized clinical trial of a 3-month, 12-dose regimen of a combination of rifapentine and isoniazid. JAMA Pediatr 2015; 169(3): 247-55. [http://dx.doi.org/10.1001/jamapediatrics.2014.3158] [PMID: 25580725]

[13]   Borisov AS, Bamrah Morris S, Njie GJ, *et al.* Update of Recommendations for Use of Once-Weekly Isoniazid-Rifapentine Regimen to Treat Latent *Mycobacterium tuberculosis* Infection. MMWR Morb Mortal Wkly Rep 2018; 67(25): 723-6. [http://dx.doi.org/10.15585/mmwr.mm6725a5] [PMID: 29953429]

[14]   Den Boon S, Matteelli A, Ford N, Getahun H. Continuous isoniazid for the treatment of latent tuberculosis infection in people living with HIV. AIDS 2016; 30(5): 797-801. [http://dx.doi.org/10.1097/QAD.0000000000000985] [PMID: 26730567]

[15]   Swindells S, Ramchandani R, Gupta A, *et al.* BRIEF TB/A5279 Study Team. One Month of Rifapentine plus Isoniazid to Prevent HIV-Related Tuberculosis. N Engl J Med 2019; 380(11): 1001-11. [http://dx.doi.org/10.1056/NEJMoa1806808] [PMID: 30865794]

[16]   Seddon JA, Fred D, Amanullah F, *et al.* Post-exposure management of multidrug-resistant tuberculosis contacts: evidence-based recommendations Policy Brief No 1. Dubai, United Arab Emirates: Harvard Medical School Center for Global Health Delivery–Dubai 2015.

[17]   Zhang Y, Yew WW. Mechanisms of drug resistance in *Mycobacterium tuberculosis*. Int J Tuberc Lung Dis 2009; 13(11): 1320-30. [PMID: 19861002]

[18]   Alangaden GJ, Manavathu EK, Vakulenko SB, Zvonok NM, Lerner SA. Characterization of fluoroquinolone-resistant mutant strains of *Mycobacterium tuberculosis* selected in the laboratory and isolated from patients. Antimicrob Agents Chemother 1995; 39(8): 1700-3. [http://dx.doi.org/10.1128/AAC.39.8.1700] [PMID: 7486904]

CHAPTER 13

Surgical Treatment in Tuberculosis

Abstract: Despite recent advances in the pharmacologic treatment of tuberculosis, some patients are left with residual or persistent sequels that could benefit from surgical intervention.

Most experts believe that surgical treatment is rarely necessary in patients with pan-sensitive tuberculosis, and is only necessary in case of complications, such as massive hemoptysis, empyema, bronchopleural fistula, *etc.*

The main indication for surgical treatment is MDR/XDR-TB. Surgical treatment in pulmonary MDR-TB is usually indicated in patients with inadequate response to medical therapy and localized lung lesions.

Indications for surgical treatment in tuberculosis can be classified as emergency surgery, urgent surgery, and elective surgery. It is recommended, when possible, that chemotherapy should be administered for at least three months before surgery to reduce the bacillary load and reduce the risk of complications.

There are four essential criteria that a patient must fulfill to be considered as a candidate for surgery in MDR-TB:

1. The patient must have localized disease and adequate respiratory function (forced expiratory volume in one second [FEV-1] $\geq$1.5 L in cases of lobectomy and $\geq$2.0 L for pneumonectomy) that will allow the surgical removal of the lesion.

2. The mycobacterial strain causing the disease must have a complex resistant profile, a characteristic associated with a high risk of treatment failure or relapse.

3. Lung tissue, including the airway around the resection margins, should be free of disease to reduce the risk of fistula at the bronchial stump.

4. The availability of enough efficient second-line drugs for treatment after surgery.

Keywords: Emergency surgery, Fistula, Lobectomy, Pneumonectomy, Surgery, Urgent surgery.

Rafael Laniado-Laborín

INTRODUCTION

A Brief History of Surgical Treatment for Tuberculosis

The pioneer of collapse therapy for the pulmonary disease was James Carson, a Scottish physician. He described the physiological benefits of artificial pneumothorax in the year 1822. Although therapeutic pneumothorax would produce short-term improvement, it frequently had complications, and some of them were life-threatening, including empyema, respiratory failure, hemorrhage, and mediastinal shift, therefore, the procedure was abandoned [1].

Later on, John Benjamin Murphy, in 1889, stated that the lung should be forced to immobilization and physiological rest. This immobilization could be achieved through different surgical collapse interventions:

1. Artificial pneumothorax.

2. Thoracoscopy and resection of adhesions (internal pneumolysis).

3. Phrenic nerve operations.

4. Thoracoplasty: the technique of choice was the Sauerbruch paravertebral thoracoplasty in which ribs one to eleven were excised, each, from six to eight centimeters from the costotransverse articulation.

5. Extra-pleural pneumolysis (plombage): after resection of a rib, the parietal pleura is separated from the chest wall, and into the resultant extra-pleural space, a mixture of paraffin wax and bismuth was inserted [2].

It was thought at that time that since it was not possible to increase the specific resistance of the patient to tuberculosis, it was more feasible to reduce the virulence of *M. tuberculosis* by resting the lungs through immobilization by collapse [3].

Other adjuvant interventions included treatment with light. This may have been general, local, or both, and the source of light could have been solar, artificial sources like the carbon-arc lamp, or a combination of both [4, 5].

By the 1940s, collapse therapy was considered state of the art for the treatment of tuberculosis, since there was no other effective medical treatment available, and surgeons believed that for a unilateral disease, it was a procedure *"...that no longer needs defense. The problem is not, shall collapse be employed, but what form of collapse is indicated"* [6].

With the discovery of streptomycin in 1944 and other effective drugs during the next two decades, the need for surgical treatment of tuberculosis gradually diminished. However, although chemotherapy now will cure most of the cases, the appearance of drug-resistant strains represents a new challenge. Fortunately, unlike the pre-chemotherapy era, when surgery had limited success due to technical limitations, improvements in surgical and anesthetic techniques and post-operative care have dramatically reduced morbidity and mortality after surgery in tuberculosis [1].

Modern Surgical Treatment of Pulmonary Tuberculosis

Despite recent advances in the treatment of tuberculosis, some patients are left with residual or persistent sequels that could benefit from surgical intervention. Currently, complications of the disease (see Table **1**) and MDR-TB are the primary indications for surgery in pulmonary tuberculosis.

Table 1. Indications for surgery in pulmonary tuberculosis.

Indications
1. Complications and sequels of pulmonary tuberculosis (empyema, persistent pneumothorax due to bronchopleural fistula, pulmonary mycetoma in residual lung cavity, *etc.*)
2. Persistent hemoptysis (and massive hemoptysis) from cavitary disease
3. Drug-resistant tuberculosis with persistently positive sputum culture despite adequate chemotherapy in patients with localized disease or minimal disease in contralateral lung
4. Drug resistant tuberculosis with limited chemotherapy options
5. High risk of relapse based on the drug-resistance profile and radiological findings
6. Intolerable side effects or toxicity of antituberculosis drugs

Most experts believe that surgical treatment is rarely necessary (and only in case of complications such as massive hemoptysis, empyema, bronchopleural fistula, *etc.*) in patients with pan-sensitive tuberculosis. Currently, the main indication for surgical treatment is MDR/XDR-TB [7].

Surgical treatment in pulmonary MDR-TB is usually indicated in patients with inadequate response to medical therapy and localized lung lesions [1]. This, however, requires state-of-the-art technology and excellent post-operative support to be successful; unfortunately, underdeveloped countries that usually have the highest burden of drug-resistant TB lack the resources for this type of surgery. Surgical programs in developed countries with low TB burden have the technical resources but lack experience. In contrast, surgical programs in developing countries with high TB burden have lots of experience but usually very limited resources.

Tuberculosis sequelae are defined as chronic, non-active residual lesions (symptomatic or asymptomatic); these include destroyed lung, cavitary lesions, lung mycetoma, bronchiectasis, lung abscess, lung gangrene, empyema, and bronchopleural fistula [8]. Antituberculosis drugs penetrate poorly into thick-walled lung cavities that harbor high loads of mycobacteria (10^8-10^9 bacilli); this leads to treatment failure and a lack of culture conversion. The removal of this poorly perfused and severely damaged lung tissue increases the likelihood of healing with medical treatment.

One common indication for surgical treatment in tuberculosis is in patients with hemoptysis. Surgery is indicated in patients with life-threatening severe hemoptysis ($\geq$500 mL/24 hours) and in those with persisting mild or moderate hemoptysis despite adequate medical treatment. Although bronchial artery embolization can occasionally control major bleeding, its effect is only temporary, and recurrence occurs in virtually every case. Surgical resection of the bleeding lesion, usually a lobectomy to remove a bleeding lung cavity, can be curative and lifesaving, and perioperative mortality has been reported to be 7% in these cases [9].

Empyema and constrictive pleural disease might require surgical treatment if not resolved with medical management and tube thoracostomy. Sometimes, the clinical condition of the patient will not allow a major surgical procedure (*e.g.*, decortication) and an open window thoracostomy (Eloesser procedure) will help to drain the empyema and control local infection.

Patients with MDR-TB who might benefit from adjuvant surgery are those that fail to convert their cultures after six months of treatment, despite receiving an adequate drug regimen (defined as a regimen that includes at least 4 effective drugs based on drug susceptibility testing and not been used by the patient in the past). Another subset of MDR-TB patients that could benefit from adjuvant surgery are those that did convert their culture but are considered to have a high risk of relapse due to extensive residual disease.

Indications for surgical treatment in tuberculosis can be classified as emergency, urgent, and elective surgery [7]:

1. Emergency surgery: without surgery, death is imminent and unavoidable: massive hemoptysis, tension pneumothorax. Mortality with surgery is 18% compared with a 75% rate in patients treated without surgery [10].

2. Urgent: progression of the disease or recurrent hemoptysis despite an adequate antituberculosis regimen.

3. Elective: includes most cases that require surgery.
  a. localized cavitary TB with persistent positive cultures after six months of supervised treatment.

  b. MDR/XDR-TB that is failing despite adequate antituberculosis treatment.

  c. Complications and sequelae of the TB (including MDR/XDR-TB): empyema and pachypleuritis, pulmonary cavity with mycetoma, bronchopleural fistula, airway stenosis, symptomatic bronchiectasis.

The ideal time to carry out the surgery is controversial. It is recommended, when possible, that chemotherapy should be administered for at least three months before surgery to reduce the bacillary load and reduce the risk of complications [11].

In patients with a strain resistant to most available antituberculosis drugs, surgery is recommended as soon as 1-2 months after starting chemotherapy with the best possible drug regimen [12, 13]. It must be emphasized that post-operative chemotherapy must continue to complete the original estimated length, usually 18-24 months post-operatively [14].

The Success of Surgical Treatment in Pulmonary Tuberculosis

A meta-analysis and a systematic review reported a treatment success rate of surgery in MDR-TB, ranging from 84% to 92% [14, 15]. A study from South Africa reported that the cure rates of adjuvant surgery in selected patients with MDR-TB co-infected with HIV were equivalent to those of HIV negative patients and significantly higher than those with MDR-TB-HIV treated with medical therapy alone [16].

Pre-Operative Evaluation

A thorough clinical history and chest radiography, including a CT scan, sputum status (smears and cultures), hemogram, blood chemistry, arterial blood gases, and lung function tests, are essential for the pre-operative evaluation of a potential surgical candidate. An echocardiogram could be indicated to rule out pulmonary hypertension or cardiac failure. When possible, it is preferable that the patient has an adequate nutritional status and is receiving a treatment regimen that includes at least four effective drugs according to drug susceptibility testing. Pre-operative bronchoscopy is recommended to rule out endobronchial disease at the site of the planned bronchial stump.

It is essential that there is excellent communication between the treating physicians and the thoracic surgeons and that the patient is aware that in MDR/XDR-TB, surgery is an adjuvant and that it will be necessary to complete 18-24 months of antituberculosis treatment after the surgical procedure.

There are four essential criteria that a patient must fulfill to be considered as a candidate for surgery in MDR-TB [7]:

1. The patient must have localized disease and adequate respiratory function (forced expiratory volume in one second [FEV-1] ≥1.5 L in cases of lobectomy and ≥2.0 L for pneumonectomy) that will allow the surgical removal of the lesion.

2. The strain causing the disease must have a complex resistant profile, a characteristic associated with a high risk of treatment failure or relapse.

3. Lung tissue, including the airway around the resection margins, should be free of disease to reduce the risk of fistula at the bronchial stump.

4. The availability of enough efficient second-line drugs for treatment after surgery.

Unfortunately, many MDR patients and most XDR-TB patients will have extensive bilateral lesions and reduced respiratory function reserves that make the option of surgical treatment impossible.

In 2014, the WHO recommended a patient-centered approach [7]. The patients and relatives should be thoroughly explained the risks and benefits of the planned surgical procedure, and written informed consent should be obtained in every case.

The patient must be made aware of the risks/benefits and possible complications of the planned surgical procedure and the need to comply with the post-operative pulmonary physiotherapy program and the antituberculosis drug regimen for at least 18 months after the surgery.

Surgery can be performed either by open thoracotomy or video-assisted thoracoscopy. Video-assisted thoracoscopic surgery (VATS) is an alternative to open thoracotomy for surgical lobectomy in patients with tuberculosis. VATS has

several advantages, including shorter surgery time, less post-operative pain, fewer complications, and shorter post-operative hospital stay [17].

During surgery, the use of a double-lumen endotracheal tube with single lung ventilation is indispensable to prevent spillage of infected secretions into the dependent lung. When possible, anatomical resections are preferred since they are associated with better results, and special care should be taken to avoid the contamination of the pleural space while performing the resection. It is recommended to reinforce the bronchial stump with muscle flaps to prevent a bronchopleural fistula, especially in patients with positive sputum at the time of the surgery.

Resection usually will require lobectomy or pneumonectomy, and wedge or segmental resections should be avoided since they are associated with a higher rate of complications.

Resectional procedures in tuberculosis (lobectomy, pneumonectomy), unlike procedures for other diseases (*e.g.* cancer) are usually technically more difficult since, due to fibrotic tissue and calcified lymph nodes, there is more bleeding and more post-operative air leaks during dissection of bronchial structures. Table **2** shows the most common surgical procedures for pulmonary TB.

Table 2. Surgical procedures for pulmonary tuberculosis*.

Surgical Procedures
Pleura
Decortication, pleurectomy, open thoracoscopy (Eloesser procedure)
Lung
Lobectomy, bilobectomy, pneumonectomy
Bronchi: stenting, occlusion, resection, bronchoplasty, re-amputation of bronchial stump
Others
Thoracoplasty (staged, extrapleural, modified, Schede)
Muscle flap (thoracomyoplasty) with intercostal, latissimus, or serratus anterior muscle
Plombage (ping pong balls; tissue expander)
Anterior thoracic spine approach (Potts disease)

*Modified from [1].

Post-Operative Care

Ideally, initial management should be carried out in an intensive care unit. Antituberculosis drugs should be re-started as soon as possible. Depending on the amount of trans operative bleeding and the levels of hemoglobin after surgery, blood transfusions might be necessary. Pulmonary physiotherapy, including incentive spirometry, is essential to prevent atelectasis. Chest tubes are removed when drainage of fluid and air has stopped, and the remaining lung has fully expanded.

Surgery for Extrapulmonary Tuberculosis

Tuberculosis can occur at any anatomic site secondary to hematogenous dissemination. Surgical treatment for extrapulmonary tuberculosis may be necessary to establish the diagnosis of lesions of unknown etiology or to treat local complications of TB in extrapulmonary sites (*e.g.*, spinal tuberculosis) [18].

Cervical lymphadenitis (also known as scrofula) is treated with antituberculosis drugs, but it may require lymph node aspiration or biopsy to establish the diagnosis, or occasionally surgical debridement to remove necrotic soft tissue [19].

Tuberculosis of the central nervous system is a common presentation of extrapulmonary TB [20]. A tuberculosis brain abscess may require surgical drainage, and a ventriculoperitoneal shunt might be needed to treat hydrocephalus complicating tuberculosis meningitis.

Pott's disease (spinal tuberculosis) is the most common presentation of skeletal tuberculosis. It is frequently complicated by spinal cord compression and surgery will be necessary to decompress it [21].

Tuberculosis of the genitourinary system is another common complication of disseminated TB. Perinephric abscess with or without extension into the retroperitoneal space and iliopsoas muscles will sometimes require a nephrectomy and drainage [22]. In males, TB can cause prostatitis, seminal vesicle disease, and epididymitis; in females, tuberculosis can cause pelvic inflammatory disease. In both scenarios, surgery might be needed to treat complications not resolved with drug therapy [23, 24].

Tuberculosis peritonitis can be either characterized by lymphadenopathy and fibrosis of the peritoneal tissues and omentum (plastic peritonitis) or by serous peritonitis with lymphocytic ascites accumulation. Both presentations can be identified by computed tomography scanning [25]. The diagnosis will usually be established at laparotomy (or laparoscopy); biopsies will demonstrate granulomatous inflammation, and cultures will recover *M. tuberculosis*.

Ileocecal tuberculosis is the most common site of gastrointestinal TB; complications include bleeding, obstruction, and perforation. Anorectal TB is also a common complication with the presence of anal fissures, fistulas, and perirectal abscesses. Surgical intervention may be required for the management of these gastrointestinal complications [18].

REFERENCES

[1] Dewan RK, Pezzella AT. Surgical aspects of pulmonary tuberculosis: an update. Asian Cardiovasc Thorac Ann 2016; 24(8): 835-46.
[http://dx.doi.org/10.1177/0218492316661958] [PMID: 27471312]

[2] O'Shaughnessy L, Crawford JH. The surgical treatment of pulmonary tuberculosis. Postgrad Med J 1938; 14(148): 38-48.
[http://dx.doi.org/10.1136/pgmj.14.148.38] [PMID: 21313103]

[3] Davies HM. Surgical treatment in cases of pulmonary tuberculosis. BMJ 1923; 1(3239): 138-40.
[http://dx.doi.org/10.1136/bmj.1.3239.138] [PMID: 20770985]

[4] Gauvain H. Discussion on light treatment in surgical Tuberculosis. Proc R Soc Med 1927; 20(6): 807-12.
[http://dx.doi.org/10.1177/003591572702000621]

[5] Sauer PK. The treatment of surgical tuberculosis with the Carbon-arc lamp. Ann Surg 1922; 75(4): 400-3.
[http://dx.doi.org/10.1097/00000658-192204000-00003] [PMID: 17864616]

[6] Holman E, Pierson P. Selective collapse by partial thoracoplasty. Recent advances in the surgical treatment of pulmonary tuberculosis. Cal West Med 1938; 48(5): 312-7.
[PMID: 18744508]

[7] World Health Organization. The role of surgery in the treatment of pulmonary TB and multidrug- and extensively drug-resistant TB. 2014. https://www.euro.who.int/__data/assets/pdf_file/0005/259691/The-role-of-surgery-in-the-treatment-of-pulmonary-TB-and-multidrug-and-extensively-drug-resistant-TB.pdf

[8] Massard G, Olland A, Santelmo N, Falcoz PE. Surgery for the sequelae of postprimary tuberculosis. Thorac Surg Clin 2012; 22(3): 287-300.
[http://dx.doi.org/10.1016/j.thorsurg.2012.05.006] [PMID: 22789594]

[9] Erdogan A, Yegin A, Gürses G, Demircan A. Surgical management of tuberculosis-related hemoptysis. Ann Thorac Surg 2005; 79(1): 299-302.
[http://dx.doi.org/10.1016/j.athoracsur.2004.05.016] [PMID: 15620962]

[10] Yablonskii PK, Kudriashov GG, Avetisyan AO. Surgical resection in the treatment of pulmonary tuberculosis. Thorac Surg Clin 2019; 29(1): 37-46.
[http://dx.doi.org/10.1016/j.thorsurg.2018.09.003] [PMID: 30454920]

[11] Bai L, Hong Z, Gong C, Yan D, Liang Z. Surgical treatment efficacy in 172 cases of tuberculosis-destroyed lungs. Eur J Cardiothorac Surg 2012; 41(2): 335-40.
[http://dx.doi.org/10.1016/j.ejcts.2011.05.028] [PMID: 21684172]

[12] Pomerantz BJ, Cleveland JC Jr, Olson HK, Pomerantz M. Pulmonary resection for multi-drug resistant tuberculosis. J Thorac Cardiovasc Surg 2001; 121(3): 448-53.
[http://dx.doi.org/10.1067/mtc.2001.112339] [PMID: 11241079]

[13] Shiraishi Y, Katsuragi N, Kita H, Tominaga Y, Kariatsumari K, Onda T. Aggressive surgical treatment of multidrug-resistant tuberculosis. J Thorac Cardiovasc Surg 2009; 138(5): 1180-4.
[http://dx.doi.org/10.1016/j.jtcvs.2009.07.018] [PMID: 19837220]

[14] Xu HB, Jiang RH, Li L. Pulmonary resection for patients with multidrug-resistant tuberculosis: systematic review and meta-analysis. J Antimicrob Chemother 2011; 66(8): 1687-95.
[http://dx.doi.org/10.1093/jac/dkr210] [PMID: 21642292]

[15] Marrone MT, Venkataramanan V, Goodman M, Hill AC, Jereb JA, Mase SR. Surgical interventions for drug-resistant tuberculosis: a systematic review and meta-analysis. Int J Tuberc Lung Dis 2013; 17(1): 6-16.
[http://dx.doi.org/10.5588/ijtld.12.0198] [PMID: 23232000]

[16]   Alexander GR, Biccard B. A retrospective review comparing treatment outcomes of adjuvant lung resection for drug-resistant tuberculosis in patients with and without human immunodeficiency virus co-infection. Eur J Cardiothorac Surg 2016; 49(3): 823-8.
[http://dx.doi.org/10.1093/ejcts/ezv228] [PMID: 26142471]

[17]   Han Y, Zhen D, Liu Z, *et al.* Surgical treatment for pulmonary tuberculosis: is video-assisted thoracic surgery "better" than thoracotomy? J Thorac Dis 2015; 7(8): 1452-8.
[http://dx.doi.org/10.3978/j.issn.2072-1439.2015.08.08] [PMID: 26380771]

[18]   Fry DE. Extra-pulmonary tuberculosis and its surgical treatment. Surg Infect (Larchmt) 2016; 17(4): 394-401.
[http://dx.doi.org/10.1089/sur.2016.046] [PMID: 27058682]

[19]   Omura S, Nakaya M, Mori A, *et al.* A clinical review of 38 cases of cervical tuberculous lymphadenitis in Japan: The role of neck dissection. Auris Nasus Larynx 2016; pii: S0385-146(16): 30025-6.
[http://dx.doi.org/10.1016/j.anl.2016.01.002.]

[20]   Schaller MA, Wicke F, Foerch C, Weidauer S. Central nervous system tuberculosis : etiology, clinical manifestations and neuroradiological features. Clin Neuroradiol 2019; 29(1): 3-18.
[http://dx.doi.org/10.1007/s00062-018-0726-9] [PMID: 30225516]

[21]   Hogan JI, Hurtado RM, Nelson SB. Mycobacterial musculoskeletal infections. Thorac Surg Clin 2019; 29(1): 85-94.
[http://dx.doi.org/10.1016/j.thorsurg.2018.09.007] [PMID: 30454925]

[22]   Daher EdeF, da Silva GB Jr, Barros EJ. Renal tuberculosis in the modern era. Am J Trop Med Hyg 2013; 88(1): 54-64.
[http://dx.doi.org/10.4269/ajtmh.2013.12-0413] [PMID: 23303798]

[23]   Kulchavenya E, Zhukova I, Kholtobin D. Spectrum of urogenital tuberculosis. J Infect Chemother 2013; 19(5): 880-3.
[http://dx.doi.org/10.1007/s10156-013-0586-9] [PMID: 23526041]

[24]   Neonakis IK, Spandidos DA, Petinaki E. Female genital tuberculosis: a review. Scand J Infect Dis 2011; 43(8): 564-72.
[http://dx.doi.org/10.3109/00365548.2011.568523] [PMID: 21438789]

[25]   Suri S, Gupta S, Suri R. Computed tomography in abdominal tuberculosis. Br J Radiol 1999; 72(853): 92-8.
[http://dx.doi.org/10.1259/bjr.72.853.10341698] [PMID: 10341698]

BCG Vaccination

Abstract: The BCG vaccine is derived from the *Bacillus Calmette-Guérin* (BCG) and is the most utilized vaccine in the history of humankind. Calmette and Guérin developed it in the Pasteur Institute from an original strain of *Mycobacterium bovis*.

The use of BCG vaccine is limited to the prevention of disseminated and meningeal TB, the most severe forms of the disease in children. BCG vaccination is recommended in countries or settings with a high incidence of TB. A single dose of BCG vaccine should be given to all healthy neonates at birth. The standard dose of BCG vaccine is 0.05 mL for infants aged less than one year and 0.1 mL for those aged one year and older. Studies have shown minimal or no evidence of additional benefits of repeat BCG vaccination against TB.

BCG vaccination is not recommended during pregnancy and it is contraindicated for individuals with immunodeficiency. HIV-infected children, when vaccinated with BCG at birth, are at increased risk of developing disseminated BCG disease.

An effective vaccine preventing pulmonary TB in adults is urgently needed but has long been considered by the TB community as an elusive goal. The slight decrease in the global incidence of TB and the rise in multidrug-resistant TB (MDR-TB) are elements that show the critical state of the TB epidemic and emphasize the need for the development of new tools, including candidates for an effective vaccine.

Keywords: BCG, Disseminated disease, HIV, Meningitis, Vaccination.

INTRODUCTION

Currently, the BCG vaccine is the only tuberculosis (TB) vaccine recommended and included in the calendar of the World Health Organization (WHO) vaccination for countries with a high incidence of TB. This vaccine, derived from the *Bacillus Calmette-Guérin* (BCG), is the most utilized in the history of humankind and has been used since 1921 to save millions of lives [1]. Calmette and Guérin developed it in the Pasteur Institute from an original strain of *Mycobacterium bovis* [2].

Protection against TB from the BCG vaccine is limited to the most severe forms of TB in children, *i.e.*, disseminated and meningeal TB [3].

Rafael Laniado-Laborín

Unfortunately, the protection from BCG in the general population ranges between 0 and 80%. This considerable variation is related to several factors, such as genetic differences in the BCG strains used for immunization, environmental influences, and host factors [2, 4].

WHO RECOMMENDATIONS FOR BCG VACCINATION [5]

BCG vaccination is recommended in countries or settings with a high incidence of TB. A single dose of BCG vaccine should be administered to all healthy neonates at birth for prevention of TB. If the BCG vaccine cannot be given at birth, it should be given at the earliest opportunity thereafter and should not be delayed in order to protect the child before exposure to infection occurs.

The standard dose of BCG vaccine is 0.05 mL for infants aged less than one year and 0.1 mL for those aged one year and older. BCG vaccines must be administered by intradermal injection, and a bleb formation can verify correct intradermal administration. The vaccine should be given in the lateral aspect of the upper arm.

Countries with a low incidence of TB may choose to vaccinate neonates selectively in groups at high risk for TB. High-risk groups include the following:

a. Neonates born to parents (or other close contacts/relatives) with current or previous TB.

b. Neonates born in households with contacts to countries with a high incidence of TB.

c. Neonates in any other locally identified risk group with TB.

In older unvaccinated children who have tested negative for infection (tuberculin skin test or IFN-γ release assays), BCG vaccination is also indicated.

BCG vaccination may also be indicated in unvaccinated not infected individuals at risk of occupational exposure: *e.g.*, health-care workers, laboratory workers, medical students, prison workers, *etc.*)

Studies have shown minimal or no evidence of any additional benefit of repeat BCG vaccination against TB [6]. Therefore, revaccination is not recommended even if the TST reaction or result of an IGRA is negative.

BCG vaccination is not recommended during pregnancy, and it is contraindicated for individuals with immuno deficiency (*e.g.*, HIV/AIDS, congenital immuno deficiency, leukemia, lymphoma or other malignant diseases) and for patients undergoing immunosuppressive treatment. Infants exposed to immunosuppressive therapy in the uterus or *via* breastfeeding should not receive BCG vaccination.

Children who are HIV-infected when vaccinated with BCG at birth are at increased risk of developing disseminated BCG disease. However, if HIV-infected individuals, including children receiving antiretroviral therapy (ART), are clinically well and immunologically stable (CD4% >25% for children aged five years), they should be vaccinated with BCG.

A vaccine preventing pulmonary TB in adults is obviously needed but has long been considered by the TB community as an elusive goal. The WHO End TB Strategy has set ambitious targets for the elimination of tuberculosis but present trends suggest that the researchers will not be able to meet those goals by the projected deadline [7]. Our current approaches are insufficient, and we urgently need research for the development of new tools. The slow decrease in the global incidence of TB and the upsurge in multidrug-resistant TB (MDR-TB) are elements that show the critical state of the TB epidemic and emphasize the need for the development of new tools, including candidates for a vaccine. Health modeling has demonstrated the added value of a vaccine that could prevent pulmonary TB in adults [8].

So far, at least 13 new vaccines intended to prevent infection (pre-exposure), the progression of the disease, and the reactivation of latent infection by TB (post-exposure) are in different stages of evaluation but still far from a clinical application [1].

Recently, results from a placebo-controlled trial for the administration of an experimental BCG vaccine (M72/AS01E) in adults infected with *M. tuberculosis* (defined as a positive result on interferon-γ release assay) without evidence of active disease, were obtained in three African countries. The primary objective was to evaluate the efficacy of M72/AS01E to prevent active pulmonary tuberculosis disease, according to the first case definition (bacteriologically confirmed pulmonary tuberculosis not associated with human immuno deficiency virus infection). Participants were followed for 3 years. Among the 3,289 participants, 13 of the 1,626 participants in the M72/AS01E group, as compared to 26 of the 1,663 participants in the placebo group, had cases of tuberculosis (incidence, 0.3 *vs.* 0.6 cases per 100 person-years). The vaccine efficacy at month 36 was 49.7% (90% CI, 12.1 to 71.2; 95% CI, 2.1 to 74.2). Serious adverse events, potential immune-mediated diseases, and deaths occurred with similar frequencies in the two groups. These results are interesting since the vaccine was administered to individuals already infected with *M. tuberculosis* [9].

REFERENCES

[1] Muñiz-Salazar R, Laniado-Laborín R. La tuberculosis en México. Editorial UABC. 317-22. ISBN 978-607-607-518-0.

[2] Liu J, Tran V, Leung AS, Alexander DC, Zhu B. BCG vaccines: their mechanisms of attenuation and impact on safety and protective efficacy. Hum Vaccin 2009; 5(2): 70-8.
[http://dx.doi.org/10.4161/hv.5.2.7210] [PMID: 19164935]

[3] Trunz BB, Fine P, Dye C. Effect of BCG vaccination on childhood tuberculous meningitis and miliary tuberculosis worldwide: a meta-analysis and assessment of cost-effectiveness. Lancet 2006; 367(9517): 1173-80.
[http://dx.doi.org/10.1016/S0140-6736(06)68507-3] [PMID: 16616560]

[4] Lahey T, von Reyn CF. *Mycobacterium bovis* BCG and newvaccines for the prevention of tuberculosis. Microbiol Spectr 2016 Oct; 4(5).
[http://dx.doi.org/10.1128/microbiolspec.TNMI7-0003-2016] [PMID: 27763257]

[5] WHO Report BCG vaccine: WHO position paper, February 2018 – Recommendations World Health Organization. Vaccine 2018; 36(4): 3408-10.
[http://dx.doi.org/10.1016/j.vaccine.2018.03.009]

[6] Rodrigues LC, Pereira SM, Cunha SS, et al. Effect of BCG revaccination on incidence of tuberculosis in school-aged children in Brazil: the BCG-REVAC cluster-randomised trial. Lancet 2005; 366(9493): 1290-5.
[http://dx.doi.org/10.1016/S0140-6736(05)67145-0] [PMID: 16214599]

[7] Vekemans J, O'Brien KL, Farrar J. Tuberculosis vaccines: Rising opportunities. PLoS Med 2019; 16(4): e1002791.
[http://dx.doi.org/10.1371/journal.pmed.1002791] [PMID: 31013268]

[8] Tait DR, Hatherill M, Van Der Meeren O, et al. Systematic review of mathematical models exploring the epidemiological impact of future TB vaccines. Hum Vaccin Immunother 2016; 12(11): 2813-32.
[http://dx.doi.org/10.1080/21645515.2016.1205769] [PMID: 27448625]

[9] Tait DR, Hatherill M, Van Der Meeren O, et al. Final analysis of a trial of M72/AS01E vaccine to prevent tuberculosis. N Engl J Med 2019; 381(25): 2429-39.
[http://dx.doi.org/10.1056/NEJMoa1909953] [PMID: 31661198]

CHAPTER 15

Tuberculosis Infection Prevention and Control

Abstract: One of the main components of the End TB Strategy is the need for infection prevention and control (IPC) in health facilities and other settings where the risk of transmission is high. The strategy has three components that should be implemented as an integrated package of IPC interventions to prevent *M. tuberculosis* transmission. The main components of the policy are a) administrative controls, b) environmental controls, and c) respiratory protection. The administrative controls include the triage of patients with signs or symptoms or with known TB disease, the isolation of patients with presumed or demonstrated TB, and the prompt initiation of effective antituberculosis treatment for patients diagnosed with tuberculosis. The environmental controls include the use of upper-room germicidal ultraviolet (GUV) and natural o mechanical ventilation systems to reduce the concentration of infectious particles in the air. Finally, the respiratory protection strategy recommends using particulate respirators integrated as a part of a respiratory protection protocol.

Another essential component of the strategy is the periodic screening of all health workers with a risk of exposure to tuberculosis patients.

Keywords: Administrative controls, Environmental controls, Infection prevention, N95 masks, Respiratory protection, UV lights, Ventilation.

INTRODUCTION

The WHO End TB strategy proposed by the World Health Assembly [1] calls for a 90% reduction in TB deaths and an 80% decrease in the TB incidence rate by the year 2030. One of the main components of this strategy is the need for prevention, including infection prevention and control (IPC) in health facilities and other settings where the risk of transmission is high. These practices are aimed at reducing the concentration of infectious droplet nuclei in the air and the exposure of susceptible individuals.

Healthcare workers (HCWs) in countries with high tuberculosis prevalence are at increased risk of tuberculosis infection; unfortunately, tuberculosis infection control measures are often poorly implemented [2]. Transmission of *M. tuberculosis* is a risk in healthcare settings, and the magnitude of the risk varies by setting, occupational group, the prevalence of TB in the community, and effectiveness of TB infection-control strategy [3].

Rafael Laniado-Laborín

A recent systematic review and meta-analysis reported an overall prevalence of latent tuberculosis infection (LTBI) of 57% among all types of health care workers, but it can be as high as 64% in some countries [4].

The risk for active tuberculosis disease in HCWs is much higher than that of the general population, with rates ranging between 25 and 5,361 per 10^5 per year, depending on the working location and occupational category [5].

Although these occupational risks cannot be eliminated entirely, the implementation of well-structured prevention programs can reduce this risk to a minimum.

The infection prevention and control strategies have three components that must be implemented as an integrated package of interventions to prevent *M. tuberculosis* transmission. The elements are a) administrative controls, b) environmental controls, and c) respiratory protection [6]. There is, however, the need for managerial control for the oversight of these policies, ensuring that management structures and tools are established to support the implementation of the three mentioned levels of protection [2]. Interrupting the transmission of *M. tuberculosis* is vital to achieving the elimination of the disease. It is necessary to rapidly identify the source case and stop person-to-person transmission by reducing the concentration of infectious particles in the air and the exposure of susceptible individuals. Unfortunately, IPC practices are not routinely or systematically implemented, especially in settings with limited resources, which have the highest burden of TB and, consequently, the highest risk of transmission.

The WHO 2019 [6] recommendations for IPC are:

ADMINISTRATIVE CONTROLS

Recommendation 1: *triage patients with signs or symptoms or with known TB disease to reduce transmission of M. tuberculosis to health workers (including those in the community) and other persons attending health care facilities.*

Protocols should be implemented and enforced to identify promptly, separate from others, and manage persons who have suspected or confirmed infectious TB disease. When taking the medical history, patients should be routinely asked about a history of TB exposure, infection or disease, symptoms and signs suggestive of TB disease, and the presence of medical conditions that increase the risk of tuberculosis [3].

Recommendation 2: *Isolate (or at least separate) patients with presumed or demonstrated pulmonary or laryngeal TB to reduce transmission of M. tuberculosis to health workers and other persons attending health care facilities.*

Recommendation 3: *prompt initiation of effective antituberculosis treatment for patients diagnosed with tuberculosis to reduce transmission of M. tuberculosis to health workers (including those in the community) and other persons attending health care facilities.*

Recommendation 4: *encourage respiratory hygiene* (including cough etiquette) for patients with presumed or demonstrated pulmonary or laryngeal TB to reduce transmission of M. tuberculosis to health workers (including those in the community) and other persons attending health care facilities.*

*A surgical or procedure mask worn by the patient will significantly reduce the dissemination of infectious droplets. Patients should be instructed to keep the mask on and to change it if it becomes wet.

ENVIRONMENTAL CONTROLS

Recommendation 5: *the use of upper-room germicidal ultraviolet (GUV) systems is recommended to reduce transmission of M. tuberculosis to health workers and other persons attending health care facilities or other persons in settings with a high risk of transmission.*

Recommendation 6: *Ventilation systems, including natural, mixed-mode, mechanical ventilation, and recirculated air through high-efficiency particulate air [HEPA] filters*, are recommended to reduce M. tuberculosis transmission to health workers, persons attending health care facilities or other persons in settings with a high risk of transmission.*

*Airborne Infection Isolation (AII) rooms, commonly called negative pressure rooms, are single-occupancy patient care spaces designed to isolate airborne pathogens to a safe containment area. The airflow supplied into the room is balanced with exhaust airflow to create negative differential pressure with respect to an adjacent space, usually the hallway or an anteroom. Negative pressure provides a gentle flow of air under a closed doorway and into the room so that no airborne particulates escape into nursing staff or public areas. Exhaust from these rooms is not recirculated in the hospital ventilation system. Instead, exhaust air typically moves into dedicated ductwork that has GUV lamps and HEPA filters to make the resulting air safe; finally, the air from the room is directed into ventilation stacks on the rooftop.

RESPIRATORY PROTECTION

Recommendation 7: *Particulate respirators*, integrated as part of a respiratory protection program, are recommended to reduce M. tuberculosis transmission to health workers, persons attending health care facilities or other persons in settings with a high risk of transmission.*

*The minimum respiratory protection device is a filtering face respirator (*e.g.*, an N95 disposable respirator). The respirator must meet the minimum filtration performance for respiratory protection in areas in which patients with suspected or confirmed TB disease might be encountered. A fit test should be conducted to determine which respirator fits the user adequately and to ensure that the user knows when the respirator fits properly.

TB Screening of Health Care Workers [3]

1. All Health Care Workers (HCWs) should receive a baseline TB screening upon hire to detect infection using either a two-step* tuberculin skin test (TST) or an interferon-gamma release assay (IGRA) to test for infection with *M. tuberculosis*.

   ○ Two-step test: two tests performed within one to four weeks of each other when the initial test is negative since a single TST may elicit little immune response yet stimulate an anamnestic immune response. The second TST will elicit a much greater response and a positive reaction. It is important to detect the booster effect, as it could be confused with a new TB infection.

2. HCWs should receive TB screening annually: symptom screen for all HCWs and testing for infection with *M. tuberculosis* for those with baseline negative test results. HCWs should be instructed to report TB symptoms immediately to the occupational health unit.

3. Those with a baseline positive or newly positive test for *M. tuberculosis* infection should receive a chest radiograph to exclude TB disease.

4. Treatment of latent TB infection should be considered according to international guidelines (see chapter 12: Diagnosis and Treatment of latent TB infection).

HCWs in Tuberculosis Laboratories

Personnel that works with specimens potentially containing mycobacteria should be thoroughly trained in protocols that minimize the generation of aerosols and undergo periodic quality control testing. The risk of transmission of *M. tuberculosis* in the laboratory includes aerosol generation during manipulation of specimens and accidental percutaneous inoculation [3].

REFERENCES

[1]   WHO. The End TB Strategy: global strategy and targets for tuberculosis prevention, care and control after 2015. Geneva: World Health Organization 2015.

[2]   Verkuijl S, Middelkoop K. Protecting Our Front-liners: Occupational Tuberculosis Prevention Through Infection Control Strategies. Clin Infect Dis 2016; 62 (Suppl. 3): S231-7.
       [http://dx.doi.org/10.1093/cid/civ1184] [PMID: 27118852]

[3]   Jensen PA, Lambert LA, Iademarco MF, Ridzon R. Guidelines for preventing the transmission of *Mycobacterium tuberculosis* in health-care settings, 2005. MMWR Recomm Rep 2005; 54(RR-17): 1-141, 13, 23.
       [PMID: 16382216]

[4]   Nasreen S, Shokoohi M, Malvankar-Mehta MS. Prevalence of latent tuberculosis among health care workers in high burden countries: a systematic review and meta-analysis. PLoS One 2016; 11(10)e0164034
       [http://dx.doi.org/10.1371/journal.pone.0164034] [PMID: 27711155]

[5]   Joshi R, Reingold AL, Menzies D, Pai M. Tuberculosis among health-care workers in lowand middle-income countries: A systematic review. PLoS Med 2006; 3(12): e494.
       [http://dx.doi.org/10.1371/journal.pmed.]

[6]   WHO. guidelines on tuberculosis infection prevention and control, 2019 update. Geneva: World Health Organization 2019. License: CC BY-NC-SA 3.0 IGO.

CHAPTER 16

Antituberculosis Drugs Adverse Effects

Abstract: The treatment of tuberculosis requires the use of multiple drugs for prolonged periods, and most patients will, at some time, experience some difficulty tolerating them. In general, it is considered that there is an underestimation of the frequency of adverse effects during the treatment of tuberculosis. Although treatment of drug-sensitive disease with first-line drugs is usually well-tolerated, treatment of multidrug-resistant disease (MDR-TB) requires the use of drugs known as "second-line" drugs, which are associated with a higher frequency and severity of adverse reactions to antituberculosis drugs.

Since it is impossible to predict the response of a given patient, the use of a drug should not be avoided in advance, for fear of an adverse reaction. There are factors that influence the development of adverse reactions, including errors in the dosage of medications, genetic factors, the age of the subject (more frequent in patients older than 60 years), consumption of alcohol and illicit substances, renal failure or hepatic disease, and co-infection with HIV.

Everything possible must be done to facilitate tolerance to medicines; patients must be assured that, while side effects are inevitable, they will be treated as vigorously as possible.

This chapter discusses the adverse effects of antituberculosis drugs on different body systems and organs.

Keywords: Adverse effects, Antituberculosis, Dosage, Drugs, Hepatotoxicity, Nephrotoxicity, Neurotoxicity, Stevens-Johnson.

INTRODUCTION

The treatment of tuberculosis requires the use of multiple drugs for prolonged periods, and most patients will, at some time, experience some difficulty in tolerating them.

According to the World Health Organization, an adverse reaction to a drug is defined as "*any unintentional harmful reaction that appears at doses normally used in humans for prophylaxis, diagnosis or treatment or to modify physiological functions.*"

Primary antituberculosis drugs (isoniazid, ethambutol, rifampicin, and pyrazinamide) are generally well tolerated [1]. However, in general, it is considered that there is an underestimation of the frequency of adverse effects during the treatment of tuberculosis. Most of the reports on adverse effects in patients under treatment for tuberculosis consist of retrospective studies, not explicitly designed to evaluate the incidence of these events. The problem of Adverse Reactions to Antituberculosis Drugs (ARADs) is even more frequent in patients infected with drug-resistant *Mycobacterium tuberculosis*. The treatment of multidrug-resistant tuberculosis (MDR-TB) requires the use of drugs known as "second-line" drugs, which are associated with a higher frequency and severity of ARADs. The ARADss associated with the treatment are even more frequent in patients with extensively resistant tuberculosis (XDR-TB) and frequently require the interruption of treatment, negatively impacting the conversion of the culture and the outcome of treatment. Most patients with MDR-TB or XDR-TB live in countries with limited resources and without access to laboratory monitoring, which makes it difficult to detect some adverse effects (hearing loss, renal failure, hypothyroidism, *etc.*).

The ARADS can be divided into two broad groups. Type A reactions are the most frequent and predictable and are dose-dependent. Type B reactions are unpredictable, independent of dose, and include 15% to 20% of all ARADSs. The latter include the reactions of hypersensitivity to drugs mediated immunologically and non-immunologic idiosyncratic reactions.

According to their severity, the ARADs can be classified into two types: minor ARADs that are reported in up to 20% of the cases, and that due to their severity only require symptomatic treatment without the need to modify treatment, and severe ARADs, fortunately, less frequent (reported in less than 10% of cases) that require, in addition to symptomatic treatment, modification or even interruption of antituberculosis treatment.

However, since it is impossible to predict the response of a given patient, the use of some drugs should not be avoided in advance for fear of an adverse reaction. Most patients can tolerate complex regimens for the treatment of drug-resistant TB despite the presence of ARADs. On the contrary, some patients will have severe difficulties tolerating even relatively simple regimens with first-line drugs.

There are factors that influence the development of ARADs, including errors in the dosage of medications, genetic factors (slow acetylators), the age of the subject (more frequent in patients older than 60 years), consumption of alcohol and illicit substances, renal failure, hepatic disease and co-infection with HIV.

It is essential before starting treatment to discuss with the patient the benefits and risks associated with treatment since the patient must be fully aware of the importance of being treated. The patient must understand the need to receive a full treatment regimen and the importance of each medication included in the regimen, as well as the possible side and toxic effects associated with each one of them. Patients must be mentally prepared to tolerate the discomfort of the side effects associated with such prolonged treatment.

Everything possible must be done to facilitate tolerance to medicines; patients must be assured that, while side effects are inevitable, they will be treated as vigorously as possible. The patient must rationalize that if there were a need for retreatment in the future for having abandoned the regimen, this would surely be more toxic and less effective.

The patient should be instructed to inform the health personnel about the appearance of ARADs as soon as possible, and health personnel (health promotor, nurse, clinician) must respond quickly to the symptoms referred by the patient; careful evaluation of them will allow determining at times if these symptoms are attributable to other causes and not a manifestation of side effects or toxicity of the drugs [2].

Most patients will agree to continue with the regimen, despite the ARADs, if they understand the benefits of treatment, they are aware that tolerance develops to most of these effects after a few weeks, and they are confident that everything necessary will be done to evaluate and treat the ARADs if they arise.

SIDE AND ADVERSE EFFECT BY BODY SYSTEM

Gastrointestinal Effects

They are usually the first to appear at the start of treatment, with nausea and vomiting being the most common; occasionally, abdominal colic pain is a complaint. *It is important to remember that nausea and vomiting may also be due to hepatotoxicity*. Ethionamide is associated with nausea, vomiting, and metallic taste, which causes anorexia that can aggravate weight loss and malnutrition. PAS is also associated with nausea, vomiting, and diarrhea. The patient should have monthly liver function tests to rule out hepatoxicity. Fractioning the dose to a couple of doses per day may improve tolerance to these drugs. An antiemetic (chlorpromazine, ondansetron, domperidone, *etc.*) or a pro-kinetic agent (for example, metoclopramide) may be used 30 minutes before administering the dose of the medication and subsequently by schedule if required; the use of antacids or sucralfate (and dairy products) should be avoided in the two hours before and after administration of the fluoroquinolones as they interfere with absorption. If infection with *Helicobacter pylori* is confirmed, it should be treated as it may aggravate the digestive symptomatology. The effect of treating these adverse effects should be evaluated. If they persist and interfere with nutrition (and in the case of vomiting with inadequate absorption of other oral medications), you may have to stop the offending drug and replace it with another. Hospitalizing the patient for administration of intravenous antiemetic therapy and hydration can help in some instances.

Diarrhea secondary to PAS usually subsides after a few weeks and does not require drug discontinuation. It is recommended to start with half the dose and increase the total dose over the first two weeks to reduce the likelihood of diarrhea. Linezolid, the fluoroquinolones, and clofazimine may also be associated with nausea/vomiting, but since they are a crucial element in the treatment of MDR-TB and their bactericidal activity is dose-dependent, the dosage of these drugs should NOT be reduced [24].

Fluoroquinolones can also cause diarrhea [3]. The administration of lactobacilli or foods such as yogurt (this should be avoided within two hours of administering the fluoroquinolones as they hinder absorption) can improve bowel habits by replenishing the normal intestinal flora. The use of antidiarrheals such as loperamide is only recommended for intermittent use.

If present, treatment for gastritis and gastroesophageal reflux should be instituted. Proton pump inhibitors may be useful, but it is recommended to use them at night, as far as possible from the administration of the antituberculosis regimen, since modifying the gastric pH can modify the absorption of antituberculosis drugs. As mentioned, avoid the use of antacids and sucralfate (as well as dairy products) at least two hours before and two hours after the intake of fluoroquinolones as they interfere with their absorption.

Hepatoxicity

Drug-induced liver injury constitutes a clinical diagnosis of exclusion. In its presence, other causes of hepatitis, such as alcohol abuse or hepatitis of viral origin (especially hepatitis B or C virus infection) must be investigated methodically in subjects with risk factors [4].

There are several antituberculosis drugs with hepatotoxicity potential, including isoniazid, rifampin, pyrazinamide, ethionamide/prothionamide, PAS, moxi-floxacin, and bedaquiline. Among the first-line drugs, isoniazid is the most frequent cause of drug-associated hepatitis, but pyrazinamide, although less frequently, causes more severe liver damage. Up to 20% of subjects who receive monotherapy with isoniazid for latent tuberculosis infection experience mild and transient elevation of liver enzymes, a process known as hepatic adaptation; although any patient can develop liver damage under treatment, patients with prior liver damage are at increased risk of developing drug hepatitis. Any gastrointestinal symptoms already mentioned may occur in case of hepatotoxicity. When hepatotoxicity is suspected, all medications capable of causing liver damage should be stopped until the result of liver function tests are available. If, in doing so, the remaining regimen is very weak (less than three non-hepatotoxic active drugs) it is advisable to suspend all medications while the problem is solved in order to avoid acquisition or amplification of drug resistance. Alanine aminotransferase (ALT or TGP) is the liver enzyme more associated with hepatocellular damage secondary to antituberculosis drugs. If the liver enzymes are within normal limits, the treatment can be reinstalled with the addition of the symptomatic therapy already described for digestive complaints. ALT is more specific for liver damage than the enzyme aspartate aminotransferase (AST or TGO), which in addition to liver damage, can be elevated in case of myocardial damage, striated muscle damage or even kidney disease. When ALT is higher than AST, it suggests hepatocellular lesion by drugs. Conversely, when AST rises more than ALT, it is more suggestive of other etiologies, mainly alcohol toxicity. The differential diagnosis of elevation of transaminases, as mentioned, should include viral hepatitis B and C, especially in patients with drug dependence. When liver enzymes are elevated, but less than three times the normal upper limit (normal values: AST: 5-40 IU/L; ALT:7-56 UI/L) and not accompanied by jaundice, treatment can be continued. Even when the transaminases are only moderately elevated, the presence of jaundice (>3 mg/dL) usually indicates significant hepatocellular damage and requires the discontinuation of hepatotoxic drugs. When the liver enzymes are elevated >3 times the upper limit of normal, it is necessary to suspend the treatment and monitor the liver function tests weekly. When the enzymes decrease below two times the upper limit of normal (although if the conditions of the patient allow it, some experts recommend waiting for the liver function to normalize before restarting the treatment), potentially hepatotoxic drugs should be reintroduced one at a time. If treatment had been completely discontinued, non-hepatotoxic drugs should be introduced at the same time as the first potentially hepatotoxic drug. The patient should then be monitored clinically and perform liver function tests twice a week until he/she has taken each drug for at least a week, and their tests remain stable. A second potentially hepatotoxic medication can then be added, and the routine described is repeated as each medication is added to the regimen. If the reintroduction of a drug raises the liver enzymes again, that drug must be eliminated definitively from the regimen. Even when a drug has been identified as hepatotoxic, the rest of the drugs in the regimen must be introduced individually, as there may be more than one hepatotoxic drug. Of course, liver function tests should be monitored every month or more frequently if it is considered convenient. If pyrazinamide was one of the drugs of the original regimen, it should be definitively discontinued, given its high hepatotoxic potential [2].

Hypersensitivity and Skin Reactions

Adverse drug reactions may be manifestations confined exclusively to the skin or be part of a multisystem response associated with both first and second-line drugs. These reactions include morbilliform rashes, Stevens-Johnson syndrome, drug hypersensitivity syndrome, cutaneous vasculitis, lichenoid eruptions, and generalized exanthematous pustulosis [5].

Cutaneous ARADs typically occurs in the first weeks of treatment. In most cases, they constitute a self-limited reaction with minimal clinical consequences (for example, face and torso acne commonly associated with the use of isoniazid). Occasionally, however, cutaneous ARADs may be associated with significant morbidity and mortality (up to 30% in toxic epidermal necrolysis), requiring interruption or changes in the treatment regimen.

Patients co-infected with HIV have a higher incidence of ARADs in general and of skin ARADs in particular, including skin reactions due to hypersensitivity. Highly active antiretroviral therapy (HAART) and prophylactic treatment for *Pneumocystis jirovecii* pneumonia, which frequently are administered simultaneously with antituberculosis treatment, complicates the identification of the causative agent of the ARADs.

Morbilliform and Maculopapular Eruptions

Morbilliform reactions (measles-like) and maculopapular rashes are the most frequent adverse reactions to the skin (up to 95% of cases of cutaneous ARADs). Macular erythematous reactions with papules usually occur between one and two weeks after starting treatment. They present initially in the torso and subsequently spread peripherally. They usually disappear without the need to discontinue the antituberculosis regimen, requiring only symptomatic treatment (chlorpheniramine, hydroxyzine, or in persistent cases, low doses of prednisone). However, occasionally the maculopapular rash may be the initial manifestation of more serious reactions such as Stevens-Johnson, and drug hypersensitivity syndrome. The increase in the severity of the rash, accompanied by systemic symptoms and mucositis, are indicators of severe ARADs and require the immediate interruption of treatment.

The reactions of facial flushing or pruritus without skin rash, usually involve the face and scalp and appear 2-3 hours after the ingestion of the medications. It is usually associated with rifampicin and pyrazinamide; in general, it is mild and self-limited.

All antituberculosis medications can cause hives. The most common causative agent is isoniazid, followed by rifampicin and pyrazinamide. It has been described mainly with first-line drugs, but it can present with the use of ethionamide, cycloserine, and fluoroquinolones, and there are already reports of urticaria with linezolid and bedaquiline. The treatment should be suspended until the ARADs is resolved. If the initial reaction was not severe, and there was no evidence of anaphylaxis, try to identify the causative agent by restarting the regimen with one drug and add the remaining medicines individually.

It is necessary to consider other causes of dermatitis, such as scabies, contact dermatitis, atopic dermatitis, psoriasis, *etc*. Dry skin in diabetic patients may cause pruritus that can be treated with a moisturizing lotion. Clofazimine can also cause severe skin dryness.

Patients receiving treatment with pyrazinamide, fluoroquinolones, and especially clofazimine may present photosensitivity. They should reduce exposure to sunlight and use sunscreen lotion. This effect may persist even after the treatment has stopped.

Lichenoid Reactions

Occasionally they appear, especially in the region of the wrists, legs, and back (sometimes on the scalp and mucous membranes) as violaceous, flat, pruritic papules very similar to the lesions observed in *lichen planus*. Mucous membranes, particularly oral and genital, are the most frequently affected sites with a string-like pattern known as Wickham striae. They can disappear spontaneously, even when treatment continues. An antihistamine or low dose prednisone may be used to treat the itching. It is often difficult to identify the responsible drug because the lesions may remit slowly after the treatment is interrupted, and this effect may be secondary to several antituberculosis medicines (*e.g.*, ethambutol, isoniazid, streptomycin, and cycloserine).

Stevens-Johnson Syndrome and Toxic Epidermal Necrolysis

Sometimes dermal reactions are associated with systemic toxicity with high fever, urticaria, edema and skin and mucosal vesicles, characteristics of Stevens-Johnson syndrome (SJS), and Toxic Epidemic Necrolysis (TEN). The SJS and the TEN are considered as variants of the same condition. TEN is observed in 10% of the cases of SJS, while in TEN, the epidermal manifestations are found in more than 30% of patients.

The initial symptoms of fever, malaise, cough, burning eyes, and odynophagia are often mistaken for a viral infection of the upper respiratory tract. However, the adverse reaction progresses rapidly to epidermal necrolysis and mucositis. Painful erythema and blisters on the palms and soles are early features of SJS/NET.

It has been described during treatment with rifampicin, pyrazinamide, isoniazid, ethambutol, streptomycin, cycloserine, linezolid, and fluoroquinolones.

This reaction requires urgent hospital treatment with systemic steroids. In these cases,

TREATMENT MUST BE INTERRUPTED IMMEDIATELY IF A DRUG IS IDENTIFIED AS A CAUSE OF THIS REACTION AND IT SHOULD NOT BE USED EVER AGAIN [6]

Drug Hypersensitivity Syndrome

The drug-induced hypersensitivity syndrome has been described with several of the anti-tuberculosis drugs. Recently, patients with eosinophilia and systemic symptoms (Drug Reaction with Eosinophilia and Systemic Symptoms, or DRESS) have been described; it has been associated with the use of rifampicin, isoniazid, and ethambutol, especially if they are receiving allopurinol to treat hyperuricemia secondary to the use of pyrazinamide. In addition to the cutaneous reaction, patients have lymphadenopathy and hepatic, pulmonary, and renal involvement. The laboratory usually reveals elevated ALT and alkaline phosphatase, leukocytosis with eosinophilia (>700 cells/µL), and if there is renal involvement, renal failure. The treatment of DRESS syndrome requires the interruption of treatment until the condition resolves.

Virtually all antituberculosis drugs can cause hypersensitivity reactions; this requires, depending on the severity, to suspend all drugs until the reaction is resolved. The most frequently involved are isoniazid, ethambutol, rifampicin, pyrazinamide, ethionamide, and fluoroquinolones. If the reaction is mild and there is no evidence of anaphylaxis, angioedema, or respiratory compromise, the clinician can try to identify the responsible drug by reintroducing one drug at a time. It is recommended to start with the essential drug in the regimen unless, for some reason, it is suspected that that drug is the cause of the adverse reaction. If this is the case, desensitization can be attempted with progressively higher doses of the drug if it is tolerated; for example, if the reaction was severe, it can be started with 1/10 of the initial dose of the medicine and progressively increased. The desensitization should preferably be carried out in the hospital to be able to start treatment immediately in case of anaphylaxis. If tolerated, the drugs will have to be administered seven days a week until the end of treatment to reduce the risk of more severe reactions. *Do not attempt desensitization if the patient presented anaphylaxis or the reaction involved systemic symptoms (fever, urticaria, mucosal involvement, blisters) as occurs in Stevens-Johnson syndrome or toxic epidermal necrolysis* [7].

NEUROTOXICITY

Peripheral Neuropathy

Peripheral neuropathy is characterized by symmetric polyneuropathy with tingling, itching, and burning in the extremities. This can be followed by paresthesias, loss of ankle reflexes, and muscle weakness; patients may even develop ataxia due to loss of proprioception. The drugs most frequently involved are isoniazid, ethionamide/prothionamide, cycloserine, and linezolid. Neuropathy occurs most often in patients with diabetes, alcoholism, HIV infection, hypothyroidism, pregnancy, and malnutrition.

Isoniazid binds to pyridoxine and depletes reserves of this vitamin. Pyridoxine is required for the synthesis of γ-aminobutyric acid (GABA), the primary inhibitory neurotransmitter in the central nervous system, whose primary role is to reduce neuronal excitability. The decrease in GABA levels caused by pyridoxine deficiency has been implicated in the seizures associated with the use of isoniazid.

Peripheral neuropathy associated with isoniazid usually begins in the feet and ascends to the hands and arms, accompanied by weakness and muscle aches, and may progress to more severe symptoms such as cerebellar ataxia. The neurological examination reveals loss of sensation (to the touch, pain, position, and vibration), areflexia, muscle weakness, and atrophy.

The prophylaxis of neuropathy is carried out with pyridoxine and is usually very effective. Prophylactic treatment with 100 mg of pyridoxine should be instituted in all patients with risk factors for neuropathy and in those under treatment for MDR-TB receiving isoniazid, ethionamide/prothionamide, cycloserine, or linezolid. If neuropathy develops despite prophylaxis with B6, antineuritic treatment can be added with gabapentin, pregabalin, or carbamazepine. Linezolid neuropathy usually occurs after a few months of treatment and is dose-dependent. It often manifests with paresthesias and distal numbness in the extremities (distribution of "sock and gloves"); This effect is NOT reversible when the medication is stopped, and it does not respond to pyridoxine treatment. The initial dose of 600 mg of linezolid can be reduced to 300 or 450 mg daily, which generally allows continuing linezolid in the treatment regimen despite neuropathy [8].

EFFECTS ON THE CENTRAL NERVOUS SYSTEM (CNS)

MDR-TB, like any chronic disease, can be associated with depression; This can be mild and does not require specific treatment beyond family and health personnel support.

However, antituberculosis medications can also cause depression syndrome, especially cycloserine and ethionamide. The depression associated with cycloserine can be severe and associated with suicidal ideas. In these cases, cycloserine and ethionamide should be discontinued, and psychological support requested. In cases with severe depression, an antidepressant may be used, taking care to avoid tricyclic antidepressants in patients who are receiving linezolid due to the risk of serotonin syndrome. In patients with pre-existing depressive disorder, cycloserine should not be included in the regimen if other effective drugs are available. It should be evaluated if there is concurrent abuse of illicit substances, and request counseling support in these cases.

Cycloserine (and to a lesser extent fluoroquinolones and isoniazid) can cause psychotic outbreaks. In these cases, the entire regimen must be discontinued, and the patient must be hospitalized in a psychiatric ward for continuous surveillance and psychiatric consultation. If it had not been initially included, vitamin B6 should be added to the regimen in addition to antipsychotic medication (for example, haloperidol).

Antituberculosis drugs, especially cycloserine, fluoroquinolones, and carbapenems, can cause seizures. In the presence of seizures, the patient should be immediately hospitalized for treatment in an intensive care unit. The treatment regimen must be discontinued immediately [9, 10].

OTOTOXICITY

Toxicity on the Eighth Cranial Nerve

All antituberculosis injectables can damage the eighth cranial nerve in both its cochlear (auditory) and vestibular (balance) branches [11].

Toxicity depends directly on the total dose, which is cumulative, and its effects irreversible. Vestibular toxicity is secondary to damage to the vestibular system and is manifested by dizziness, vertigo, and loss of balance. The patient should be questioned about the presence of tinnitus or balance disorders at each monthly visit. Although other drugs can cause moderate balance disorders (cycloserine, ethionamide, fluoroquinolones, linezolid), this possibility should be considered, as well as those of other causes of balance; however, if tinnitus or balance disorders occur, they should be attributed to vestibular toxicity, and the injectable should be discontinued. This is an irreversible and intolerable adverse reaction; if the injectable is continued, the patient may be left incapacitated by vertigo or ataxia. Remember, vestibular toxicity is irreversible.

Hearing toxicity is due to damage to the cochlear branch of the eighth cranial nerve. The ototoxicity of aminoglycosides is secondary to the injury of the hairy cells of the cochlea. Initially, they affect the cells of the base of the cochlea, which affects the hearing for high frequencies; if the exposure continues, the hairy cells in the upper part of the cochlea are affected, causing hearing loss in the frequencies required for conversation, and may reach anacusis [12].

All aminoglycosides (and capreomycin) used for the treatment of drug-resistant tuberculosis are toxic to the 8th cranial nerve and can cause hearing or vestibular damage. Amikacin and kanamycin cause hearing loss more frequently than streptomycin; On the contrary, streptomycin is associated with vestibular damage more frequently than the other injectables. Capreomycin can also cause hearing loss, but the frequency seems to be less than that of the other injectables.

Virtually all patients receiving treatment with second-line injectables for drug-resistant TB experience some degree of 8th nerve damage, with decreased hearing acuity, initially experiencing loss at high frequencies. The damage should be considered irreversible. When the regimen includes an injectable, audiometry monitoring is indispensable (baseline followed by monthly examination). After sputum conversion, the injectables can be spaced 2 or 3 times a week [13].

NEPHROTOXICITY

It is estimated that up to 25% of patients treated with aminoglycosides develop nephrotoxicity.

Aminoglycosides cause kidney damage through three mechanisms:

1. Renal tubular toxicity.

2. Decreased glomerular filtration.

3. Reduction in renal blood flow.

The most important mechanism is that of renal tubular toxicity. The aminoglycosides are concentrated at the level of the proximal tubule of the nephron; once a specific concentration is reached, the aminoglycosides empty into the cytoplasm and act on the mitochondria, causing apoptosis and cell necrosis. They also inhibit the transport mechanisms of the proximal tubule, which affects the reabsorption of electrolytes. Early signs of damage are an increase in the urinary excretion of calcium, magnesium, proteins, and other organic anions, resulting in hypocalcemia, hypomagnesemia, and proteinuria [14].

Finally, aminoglycosides cause kidney damage by reducing renal blood flow through the increased resistance of the vascular bed of the kidney. This occurs after the proximal tubule has been damaged, as a compensation mechanism to prevent the loss of fluid and electrolytes.

There are several patient-specific factors that increase the risk of aminoglycoside nephrotoxicity, including advanced age, previous kidney damage, pregnancy, dehydration, renal atrophy, hypothyroidism, diabetes, hepatic dysfunction, metabolic acidosis, and sodium depletion. There are also risk factors related to the medication, including prolonged treatment duration and high cumulative doses. The concomitant use of other drugs also increases the risk, including non-steroidal anti-inflammatory drugs, loop diuretics, amphotericin B, cisplatin, cyclosporine, iodinated contrast medium, vancomycin, and cephalosporins.

All the aminoglycosides (and capreomycin) used for the treatment of tuberculosis are nephrotoxic, so a frequent and constant evaluation of renal function is required. Amikacin and kanamycin are more nephrotoxic than streptomycin. Up to one-third of patients treated with capreomycin develop an impaired renal function.

It is recommended to use a maximum dose of second-line injectable of 750 mg/day in elderly patients [15]. The calculation of the dosage of injectable drugs should be based on body weight (ideal), and if access is available, it is advisable to measure serum levels of the injectable. Aminoglycosides should be administered in a single dose per day; nephrotoxicity with this dosage is much lower than when several doses are administered per day [2].

The use of injectables can be associated with alterations in serum electrolyte levels that must be monitored monthly (potassium, chloride, sodium, calcium, magnesium). Since some antituberculosis medications can prolong the QT interval of the cardiac cycle (fluoroquinolones, especially moxifloxacin, clofazimine, delamanid, and bedaquiline), special care should be taken to maintain electrolytes levels within normal limits.

OPHTHALMOLOGICAL TOXICITY

Ethambutol is the antituberculosis drug most frequently associated with ophthalmologic toxicity. It has the potential to cause toxic optic neuropathy, with an incidence ranging from <1% at doses of 15 mg/kg to 5-6% at doses of 25 mg/kg [16]. Damage, if not detected early, might be irreversible, so monitoring is emphasized for early detection during the subclinical stage. It has been reported even after a few days of treatment, although usually it is reported after three months of treatment. Upon discovery, the drug should be discontinued immediately to prevent the progression of neuropathy and allow recovery of function. Fortunately, in most patients, the adverse effect reverts after the suspension of the medication.

Doses of 25 mg/kg are most frequently associated with damage. Ethambutol causes a retrobulbar injury of the ophthalmic nerve; the central fibers of the optic nerve are the most affected, producing blurred vision, central scotoma, and the inability to distinguish red and green colors. As the neuritis is retrobulbar, the ocular fundus examination is normal [17].

As ethambutol is eliminated by the kidney, patients with renal failure may have ophthalmologic toxicity more frequently, and the drug should be spaced, administered three times a week instead of daily, and the dose should be adjusted to the glomerular filtration rate.

It is recommended to evaluate visual acuity (Snellen test) and chromatic discrimination (Ishihara sheets) monthly. Alterations in chromatic vision (dyschromatopsia) are the most sensitive indicator of optic neuropathy. Errors in blue-yellow perception are observed in the earliest stages and errors in red-green discrimination in more advanced stages of ethambutol toxicity. These alterations occur before visual acuity and visual fields are affected.

Linezolid can also cause optic neuritis, which is also reversible. It is characterized by a progressive diminution of visual acuity and central scotomas of sudden onset with gradual loss of visual acuity and color discrimination. If there is a risk that the regimen is compromised by the suspension of linezolid, the daily dose can be reduced to 300 mg.

Other drugs (ethionamide/prothionamide, isoniazid, and clofazimine) may occasionally produce ophthalmologic toxicity.

The recommended behavior in cases with ophthalmic toxicity is to suspend the causal agent and request urgent consultation to ophthalmology [18].

Up to half of the patients treated with clofazimine may have a reddish coloration of the conjunctiva, which is dose-dependent (more noticeable at higher doses); it usually disappears after a few months of stopping the medication. In addition, clofazimine can cause pigmentary maculopathy and generalized degeneration of the retina.

Rifabutin, especially in doses> 300 mg daily, or when administered together with drugs that reduce its clearance, such as protease inhibitors, azoles, and macrolides, can cause pan-uveitis, manifested by conjunctival redness, eye pain, and loss of visual acuity. Rifabutin should be discontinued until the symptoms subside, if it is

necessary to reinstate it, it should be administered at a lower dose, ensuring that its serum levels are within the therapeutic range.

Ophthalmology should be consulted to rule out other possible etiologies of uveitis, such as HIV, bacterial, and viral infections [2].

MUSCLE AND TENDINOUS TOXICITY

Myalgias and arthralgias are frequent during antituberculosis treatment and can be caused by multiple medications (pyrazinamide, ethambutol, fluoroquinolones, isoniazid, ethionamide, and bedaquiline). The metabolite of pyrazinamide (pyrazinoic acid) inhibits the renal tubular secretion of uric acid, increasing its concentration, causing arthralgias.

Usually, it is not necessary to stop treatment, and pain is treated with nonsteroidal anti-inflammatory drugs (indomethacin, ibuprofen, or colchicine). It is convenient to rule out other causes of myalgias and arthralgias (including hypothyroidism secondary to treatment with ethionamide/prothionamide).

The terms tendinitis and tendonitis are inappropriate because, in the pathologies of the tendons, there are no inflammatory cells within the tendon. The term tendinopathy is preferred. The primary risk factor is age >60 years. Other risk factors include drug dose, preexisting tendinopathy, diabetes renal failure, and the concomitant use of glucocorticoids.

The toxicity of quinolones on the tendons is a class effect that is observed with all members of this family of synthetic antimicrobials, regardless of their route of administration and regardless of the dose used. The tendons of the lower extremities, and especially the Achilles tendon are the more frequently affected (up to 90% of cases); tendinopathy is bilateral in more than 40% of cases. Tendon rupture (especially the Achilles tendon) has been described mainly in elderly patients. Other less frequently affected sites are the rotator cuff tendon [19], the radial extensor of the carpus, the flexor tendons of the fingers of the hands and the tendon of the quadriceps (Rosa B, 2016); up to 40% of cases of tendinopathy due to quinolones are complicated by rupture of a tendon. Cases of rupture have been reported within the first two weeks of treatment, and there are reports of rupture up to six months after discontinuation of the quinolones [20].

Tendinopathy will be treated with rest and non-steroidal anti-inflammatory drugs; This adverse effect is more common with levofloxacin, so if it is possible, it can be changed to moxifloxacin. It is considered that the frequency of tendinopathy is higher with levofloxacin because it reaches high systemic concentrations, its dependence on renal elimination, and the production of toxic metabolites. Since quinolone is a generally vital element of the treatment regimen, it is unlikely that it can be discontinued.

Tendinopathy has a favorable prognosis generally within the first two months post-treatment, although recovery may take several months, and residual damage may persist in 10% of cases [21].

Table 1. Antituberculosis drugs adverse effects*.

Drug	Adverse Effect
Amikacin	Nephrotoxicity, ototxicity, vestibular toxicity, local pain with intramuscular injections, electrolyte abnormalities: hypokalemia, hypocalcemia and hypomagnesemia Should be avoided in pregnancy due to congenital deafness. Coadministration of loop diuretics and amikacin carries an increased risk of ototoxicity
Amoxicillin/clavulanate	Diarrhea and abdominal pain, nausea, vomiting, rash, hypersensitivity
Bedaquiline	QTc prolongation, hepatitis, nausea arthralgia, headache, amylase, hemoptysis, anorexia, rash Stop bedaquiline if QTc >500 ms. This effect is aggravated by low levels of magnesium and calcium Coadministration of CYP3A4 inducers (*e.g.*, rifampin, efavirenz) or inhibitors (*e.g.*, ritonavir may require dose adjustment
Clofazimine	QTc prolongation. Stop clofazimine if QTc >500 ms. Bloody stools or diarrhea, jaundice, nausea, vomiting, abdominal pain, heartburn, depression. Discoloration of skin, conjunctiva, cornea and body fluids|

(Table 1) cont.....

Drug	Adverse Effect
Delamanid	Not recommended during pregnancy. . QTc prolongation; Stop delamanid if QTc >500 ms. Nausea, vomiting, dizziness, insomnia, upper abdominal pain May cause harm to the fetus and it is not usually recommended during pregnancy
Ethambutol	Cleared by the kidney; use with caution in renal disease. Retrobulbar neuritis (dose related) and increased with simultaneous use of linezolid
Ethionamide	Should not be used during pregnancy due to teratogenicity. Nausea, vomiting, abdominal pain. Metallic taste. Hepatotoxicity. Gynecomastia, hair loss, acne, impotence, menstrual irregularities. Reversible hypothyroidism (monitor TSH). Neurotoxicity (should receive 100 mg/day of vitamin B6). Side effects may be exacerbated in patients receiving cycloserine
Imipenem/cilastatin	Diarrhea, nausea, vomiting. Seizure (in meningeal disease, especially in children)
Isoniazid	Hepatits (age-related), diarrhea, peripheral neuropathy, hypersensitivity, optic neuritis, arthralgias, drug induced lupus. Must receive vitamin B6
Levofloxacin	Arthralgias, tendon rupture (treated symptomatically) Usually avoided during pregnancy due to reports of arthropathy in animals. Requires dose adjustment in patients with renal disease. Nausea, headache, dizziness, insomnia. QTc prolongation. Stop levofloxacin if QTc >500 ms
Linezolid	Limited data in pregnancy or breastfeeding. Neuropathy (pain, numbness, weakness in extremities. Optic neuritis. Must receive vitamin B6.Anemia, thrombocytopenia Should not be administered to patients takin serotonergic drugs (such as monoamine oxidase) due to potential risk of serotonin syndrome or neuroleptic malignant syndrome
Meropenem	Diarrhea, nausea, vomiting. Seizures (less frequent compared to imipenem), hematologic toxicity, hypersensitivity
Moxifloxacin	Arthralgias, tendon rupture (treated symptomatically) Usually avoided during pregnancy due to reports of arthropathy in animals. Nausea, headache, dizziness, insomnia, hepatotoxicity. QTc prolongation, more pronounced than with levofloxacin. Stop moxifloxacin if QTc >500 ms
Para-aminosalicylate	Nausea, vomiting, diarrhea. Rare hepatotoxicity. Hematologic toxicity. Reversible hypothyroidism (increased with concomitant use of ethionamide or prothionamide
Pyrazinamide	Hyperuricemia and arthralgias. Hepatotoxicity. Photosensitivity and rash. Nausea, vomiting
Rifabutin	Leukopenia, thrombocytopenia, Rash and skin decoloration (bronzing or pseudojaundice. Anterior uveitis. Hepatotoxicity. Many drug-drug interactions (although less frequent than with rifampin). Arthralgias
Rifampin	Orange staining of body fluids. Rash and pruritus. Nausea, vomiting. Flu-like syndrome (usually with intermittent administration). Hematologic abnormalities (thrombocytopenia, hemolytic anemia)
Rifapentin	Pregnancy category C. Red-orange staining of body fluids. Rash and pruritus. Hypersensitivity. Hepatotoxicity. Hematologic abnormalities

(Table 1) cont.....

Drug	Adverse Effect
Streptomycin	Avoided in pregnancy due to congenital deafness. Nephrotoxicity (less than amikacin). Ototoxicity (increases with age). Vestibular toxicity. Local pain with IM injections. Electrolyte abnormalities, including hypokalemia, hypocalcemia and hypomagnesemia

*modified from reference [2].

THYROID TOXICITY

Ethionamide and protionamide are thionamide derivatives of nicotinic acid that are frequently used in the treatment of MDR-TB and XDR-TB (Dutta BS, 2012). Both drugs inhibit the synthesis of thyroid hormone, causing hypothyroidism, so thyroid function tests should be carried out periodically to monitor the function of this gland. This effect is due to its chemical structure, which is very similar to propylthiouracil and methimazole, drugs that inhibit the synthesis of thyroid hormone. Para-amino salicylic acid (PAS) is another second-line drug that can induce hypothyroidism. When both drugs are used simultaneously in the regimen, the risk increases considerably, with reported rates ranging from 3.5% to 28.7% [22].

Patients with HIV/AIDS and low CD4 counts are also at increased risk of hypothyroidism, perhaps because HIV infection can cause thyroid dysfunction in the presence of opportunistic infections that affect thyroid function, or secondary to thyroid infiltration by Kaposi's sarcoma. In addition, patients receiving antiretroviral treatment with stavudine, efavirenz, amprenavir, lopinavir, and ritonavir may develop hypothyroidism. If therapy with ethionamide/protionamide and/or PAS is added, the risk of hypothyroidism is theoretically higher [2].

Thyroid function tests should be requested before the start of treatment and afterward bi-monthly if the patient receives any of these medications. Hypothyroidism presents with nonspecific and vague symptoms, and can easily be missed by the clinician, especially given the wide range of common side effects in patients under treatment with second-line antituberculosis drugs.

When the TSH value is increased to 1.5 times the upper limit of normal (4.0 mlU/L), *i.e.* 10 mlU/L, replacement thyroid hormone should be added to the regimen. The usual dose ranges between 75 and 150 mcg/day, and the dosage is adjusted according to the results of follow-up thyroid function tests after two months of treatment. The goal is to normalize TSH levels [23].

HEMATOLOGICAL TOXICITY

Hematologic abnormalities during antituberculosis treatment may be due to co-morbidity (*e.g.*, renal failure, malnutrition) to disseminated tuberculous disease with involvement of the bone marrow or to the effect of antituberculosis drugs.

Drug toxicity can affect any cell line and can be due to practically any of the antituberculosis drugs, the most commonly involved being isoniazid, rifampicin, and linezolid.

Hematological reactions to isoniazid include anemia (which responds to treatment with pyridoxine), agranulocytosis, neutropenia, hemolytic anemia, disseminated intravascular coagulation, and hemophagocytic syndrome.

Thrombocytopenia is the hematological toxicity most commonly associated with the use of rifampin. This is observed more frequently in patients receiving the biweekly regimen (1-6%) than with the daily regimen (0.08%). It is considered to be an immune-mediated effect associated with antibodies against rifampicin. Thrombocytopenia is reversible if the drug is discontinued [24].

Rifampicin can also cause hemolytic anemia, mediated immunologically by antibodies; this phenomenon can be fatal if it is not detected. Rifampicin also interferes with the absorption of vitamin K and its metabolism, causing hypoprothrombinemia [8].

Linezolid causes hematological disorders by inhibiting protein synthesis at the mitochondrial level. Long courses of linezolid (>28 days) and high doses of the drug have been associated with anemia, leukopenia, thrombocytopenia, and even pancytopenia. Reversible myelosuppression and immunological mediated toxicity have been suggested as a mechanism [2].

In case of clinically significant anemia (especially with linezolid) erythrocyte counts can be increased with the use of erythropoietin if suspending the drug would jeopardize the effectiveness of the regimen.

ADVERSE CARDIOVASCULAR EFFECTS

The quinolones, in a dose-dependent effect, cause a prolongation of the QT interval by inhibition of the calcium channels (the upper limit of the corrected QT or QTc is 450 ms in men and 470 ms in women). This prolongation predisposes to *Torsades de pointes*, an arrhythmia that can be fatal. Although this effect can vary between the different agents, the prolongation is usually minimal (3-6 ms); moxifloxacin causes a more significant prolongation of QT than levofloxacin and gatifloxacin, even with daily doses of levofloxacin of 1 to 1.5 grams. However, this effect of the quinolones may be clinically significant in the presence of risk factors for *Torsades de pointes*, such as the female sex, familial long QT syndrome, other heart diseases, renal and hepatic dysfunction, electrolyte alterations and interaction with other multiple drugs that prolong the QT. In most reports of *Torsades de pointes* in patients receiving quinolone treatment, the patient was receiving other drugs that prolong QT, had hypokalemia or hypothyroidism, an entity that causes QT prolongation (and may be secondary to treatment with ethionamide/protionamide and/or PAS [25].

Bedaquiline (BDQ), a new drug for MDR/XDR-TB treatment, may prolong the QT interval, which may be associated with *Torsades de pointes*, constituting a risk for sudden death. For this reason, concomitant use of BDQ with drugs that prolong the QT interval (for example, delamanid, moxifloxacin, and to a lesser extent, levofloxacin, clofazimine, macrolides, azole antifungals, omeprazole, *etc.*) should be carefully monitored. A QTc interval >500 ms is considered as high risk and is enough reason not to initiate or suspend the BDQ and all other drugs in the regime that prolong the QT. Frequent electrocardiographic monitoring (monthly) is recommended during treatment with BDQ. Given the long half-life of the BDQ, the risk of cardiac toxicity persists even after discontinuing its use, especially if other drugs that prolong the QT interval are being administered simultaneously [26].

Delamanid (DLM), another new drug used for the treatment of MDR/XDR-TB, can also cause a prolongation of the QT interval through its main metabolite DM-6705. The clinical studies showed an increase in QTc of 14.6 ms with a dose of 200 mg daily and of 18.9 ms with a dose of 400 mg daily, reaching its maximum value at the end of the second month of treatment, without further increase later. Most patients who developed an increase in QTc had cardiovascular risk factors (including AV block and branch block) and hypokalemia. To date, there are no reports of *Torsades de pointes* or arrhythmias with the use of delamanid [27]. As in the case of the BDQ, the concomitant use of other drugs that prolong the QT (for example, bedaquiline, fluoroquinolones or clofazimine) simultaneously with DLM will have an additive effect on the QT interval, so its simultaneous use should be carefully monitored [28 - 30].

REFERENCES

[1]   Andries A, Isaakidis P, Das M, *et al.* High rate of hypothyroidism in multidrug-resistant tuberculosis patients co-infected with HIV in Mumbai, India. PLoS One 2013; 8(10): e78313.
[http://dx.doi.org/10.1371/journal.pone.0078313] [PMID: 24194919]

[2]   Curry International Tuberculosis Center and California Department of Public Health. Drug-Resistant Tuberculosis: A Survival Guide for Clinicians. 3rd ed. 2016; pp. 246-75.

[3]   Pépin J, Saheb N, Coulombe MA, *et al.* Emergence of fluoroquinolones as the predominant risk factor for Clostridium difficile-associated diarrhea: a cohort study during an epidemic in Quebec. Clin Infect Dis 2005; 41(9): 1254-60.
[http://dx.doi.org/10.1086/496986] [PMID: 16206099]

[4]   Saukkonen JJ, Cohn DL, Jasmer RM, *et al.* An official ATS statement: hepatotoxicity of antituberculosis therapy. Am J Respir Crit Care Med 2006; 174(8): 935-52.
[http://dx.doi.org/1164/rccm.200510-1666ST.]

[5]   Lehloenya RJ, Dheda K. Cutaneous adverse drug reactions to anti-tuberculosis drugs: state of the art and into the future. Expert Rev Anti Infect Ther 2012; 10(4): 475-86.
[http://dx.doi.org/10.1586/eri.12.13] [PMID: 22512756]

[6]   Miliszewski MA, Kirchhof MG, Sikora S, Papp A, Dutz JP. Stevens-johnson syndrome and toxic epidermal necrolysis: an analysis of triggers and implications for improving prevention. Am J Med 2016; 129(11): 1221-5.
[http://dx.doi.org/10.1016/j.amjmed.2016.03.022] [PMID: 27086495]

[7]   Shiohara T, Mizukawa Y. Drug-induced hypersensitivity syndrome (DiHS)/drug reaction with eosinophilia and systemic symptoms (DRESS): An update. Allergol Int 2019; pii: S1323-8930(19): 30046-2.
[http://dx.doi.org/10.1016/j.alit.2019.03.006.]

[8]   Beekmann SE, Gilbert DN, Polgreen PM. IDSA Emerging Infections Network. Toxicity of extended courses of linezolid: results of an Infectious Diseases Society of America Emerging Infections Network survey. Diagn Microbiol Infect Dis 2008; 62(4): 407-10.
[http://dx.doi.org/10.1016/j.diagmicrobio.2008.08.009] [PMID: 18929458]

[9]   Kass JS, Shandera WX. Nervous system effects of antituberculosis therapy. CNS Drugs 2010; 24(8): 655-67.
[http://dx.doi.org/10.2165/11534340-000000000-00000]

[10]   Forget EJ, Menzies D. Adverse reactions to first-line antituberculosis drugs. Expert Opin Drug Saf 2006; 5(2): 231-49.
[http://dx.doi.org/10.1517/14740338.5.2.231] [PMID: 16503745]

[11]   de Jager P, van Altena R. Hearing loss and nephrotoxicity in long-term aminoglycoside treatment in patients with tuberculosis. Int J Tuberc Lung Dis 2002; 6(7): 622-7.
[PMID: 12102302]

[12]   Lanvers-Kaminsky C, Zehnhoff-Dinnesen AA, Parfitt R, Ciarimboli G. Drug-induced ototoxicity: Mechanisms, Pharmacogenetics, and protective strategies. Clin Pharmacol Ther 2017; 101(4): 491-500.
[http://dx.doi.org/10.1002/cpt.603] [PMID: 28002638]

[13]   Arbex MA, Varella MdeC, Siqueira HR, Mello FA, de Mello FAF. Antituberculosis drugs: drug interactions, adverse effects, and use in special situations. Part 2: second line drugs. J Bras Pneumol 2010; 36(5): 641-56.
[http://dx.doi.org/10.1590/S1806-37132010000500017] [PMID: 21085831]

[14]   Peloquin CA, Berning SE, Nitta AT, *et al.* Aminoglycoside toxicity: daily *versus* thrice-weekly dosing for treatment of mycobacterial diseases. Clin Infect Dis 2004; 38(11): 1538-44.
[http://dx.doi.org/10.1086/420742] [PMID: 15156439]

[15]   Wargo KA, Edwards JD. Aminoglycoside-induced nephrotoxicity. J Pharm Pract 2014; 27(6): 573-7.
[http://dx.doi.org/10.1177/0897190014546836] [PMID: 25199523]

[16]   Kandel H, Adhikari P, Shrestha GS, Ruokonen EL, Shah DN. Visual function in patients on ethambutol therapy for tuberculosis. J Ocul Pharmacol Ther 2012; 28(2): 174-8.

[http://dx.doi.org/10.1089/jop.2011.0095] [PMID: 22136146]

[17]   Melamud A, Kosmorsky GS, Lee MS. Ocular ethambutol toxicity. Mayo Clin Proc 2003; 78(11): 1409-11.
[http://dx.doi.org/10.4065/78.11.1409] [PMID: 14601701]

[18]   Miguel A, Henriques F, Azevedo LF, Pereira AC. Ophthalmic adverse drug reactions to systemic drugs: a systematic review. Pharmacoepidemiol Drug Saf 2014; 23(3): 221-33.
[http://dx.doi.org/10.1002/pds.3566] [PMID: 24464938]

[19]   Eyer-Silva WdeA, Netto HdeB, Pinto JF, Ferry FR, Neves-Motta R. Severe shoulder tendinopathy associated with levofloxacin. Braz J Infect Dis 2012; 16(4): 393-5.
[http://dx.doi.org/10.1016/j.bjid.2012.06.015] [PMID: 22846132]

[20]   Kirchgesner T, Larbi A, Omoumi P, *et al.* Drug-induced tendinopathy: from physiology to clinical applications. Joint Bone Spine 2014; 81(6): 485-92.
[http://dx.doi.org/10.1016/j.jbspin.2014.03.022] [PMID: 24962977]

[21]   Rosa B, Campos P, Barros A, Karmali S, Gonçalves R. Spontaneous bilateral patellar tendon rupture: case report and review of fluoroquinolone-induced tendinopathy. Clin Case Rep 2016; 4(7): 678-81.
[http://dx.doi.org/10.1002/ccr3.592] [PMID: 27386128]

[22]   Satti H, Mafukidze A, Jooste PL, McLaughlin MM, Farmer PE, Seung KJ. High rate of hypothyroidism among patients treated for multidrug-resistant tuberculosis in Lesotho. Int J Tuberc Lung Dis 2012; 16(4): 468-72.
[http://dx.doi.org/10.5588/ijtld.11.0615] [PMID: 22326109]

[23]   Dutta BS, Hassan G, Waseem Q, Saheer S, Singh A. Ethionamide-induced hypothyroidism. Int J Tuberc Lung Dis 2012; 16(1): 141.
[http://dx.doi.org/10.5588/ijtld.11.0388] [PMID: 22236862]

[24]   Ramachandran G, Swaminathan S. Safety and tolerability profile of second-line anti-tuberculosis medications. Drug Saf 2015; 38(3): 253-69.
[http://dx.doi.org/10.1007/s40264-015-0267-y] [PMID: 25676682]

[25]   Khan F, Ismail M, Khan Q, Ali Z. Moxifloxacin-induced QT interval prolongation and torsades de pointes: a narrative review. Expert Opin Drug Saf 2018; 17(10): 1029-39.
[http://dx.doi.org/10.1080/14740338.2018.1520837] [PMID: 30193085]

[26]   WHO. Report of the Guideline Development Group Meeting on the use of bedaquiline in the treatment of multidrug-resistant tuberculosis, A review of available evidence (2016). Geneva: World Health Organization 2017. Licence: CC BY-NC-SA 3.0 IGO

[27]   WHO position statement on the use of delamanid for MDR-TB. Licence: CC BY-NC-SA 3.0 IGO & Gupta R, Geiter L, Hafkin J, Wells C. Delamanid and QT prolongation in the treatment of multidrug-Resistant TB. Int J Tuberc Lung Dis 2015; 19(10): 1261-2.
[http://dx.doi.org/10.5588/ijtld.15.0541] [PMID: 26459547]

[28]   Sarin R, Vohra V, Singla N, *et al.* Early efficacy and safety of Bedaquiline and Delamanid given together in a "Salvage Regimen" for treatment of drug-resistant tuberculosis. Indian J Tuberc 2019; 66(1): 184-8.
[http://dx.doi.org/10.1016/j.ijtb.2019.02.006] [PMID: 30878066]

[29]   WHO. operational handbook on tuberculosis Module 4: treatment - drug-resistant tuberculosis treatment. Geneva: World Health Organization 2020. Licence: CC BY-NC-SA 3.0 IGO.

[30]   Lan Z, Ahmad N, Baghaei P, *et al.* Collaborative Group for the Meta-Analysis of Individual Patient Data in MDR-TB treatment 2017. Drug-associated adverse events in the treatment of multidrug-resistant tuberculosis: an individual patient data meta-analysis. Lancet Respir Med 2020; 8(4): 383-94.
[http://dx.doi.org/10.1016/S2213-2600(20)30047-3] [PMID: 32192585]

SUBJECT INDEX